Zainab A.SHEHAB
Mohamed Abdel-Raheem
Hind A. A. Alahmed

Present-day imaginary stem cells and their uses in veterinary medicine

Zainab A.SHEHAB
Mohamed Abdel-Raheem
Hind A. A. Alahmed

Present-day imaginary stem cells and their uses in veterinary medicine

Noor Publishing

Imprint
Any brand names and product names mentioned in this book are subject to trademark, brand or patent protection and are trademarks or registered trademarks of their respective holders. The use of brand names, product names, common names, trade names, product descriptions etc. even without a particular marking in this work is in no way to be construed to mean that such names may be regarded as unrestricted in respect of trademark and brand protection legislation and could thus be used by anyone.

Cover image: www.ingimage.com

Publisher:
Noor Publishing
is a trademark of
Dodo Books Indian Ocean Ltd. and OmniScriptum S.R.L publishing group

120 High Road, East Finchley, London, N2 9ED, United Kingdom
Str. Armeneasca 28/1, office 1, Chisinau MD-2012, Republic of Moldova, Europe
Managing Directors: Ieva Konstantinova, Victoria Ursu
info@omniscriptum.com

Printed at: see last page
ISBN: 978-620-0-04704-5

Present-day imaginary stem cells and their uses in veterinary medicine

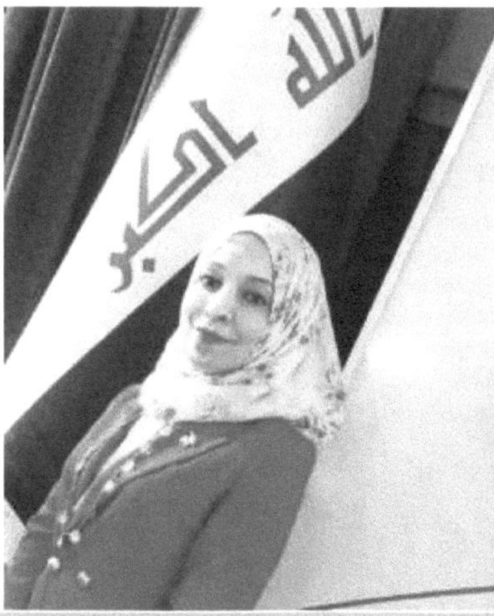

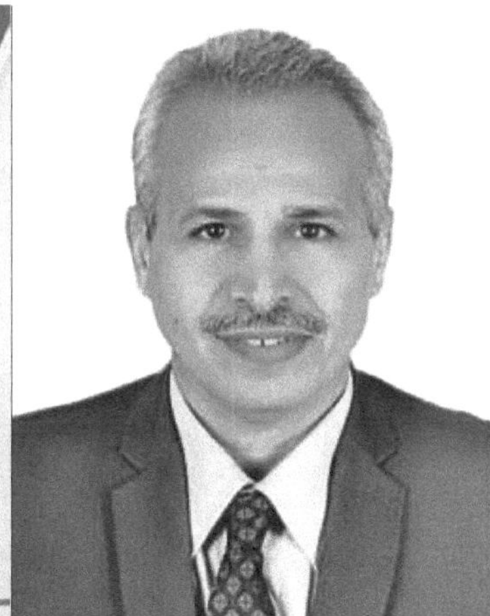

By

Assist. Prof. Dr. Zainab A.SHEHAB

Prof. Dr. Mohamed Abdel-Raheem

Dr. Hind A. A. Alahmed

(2025)

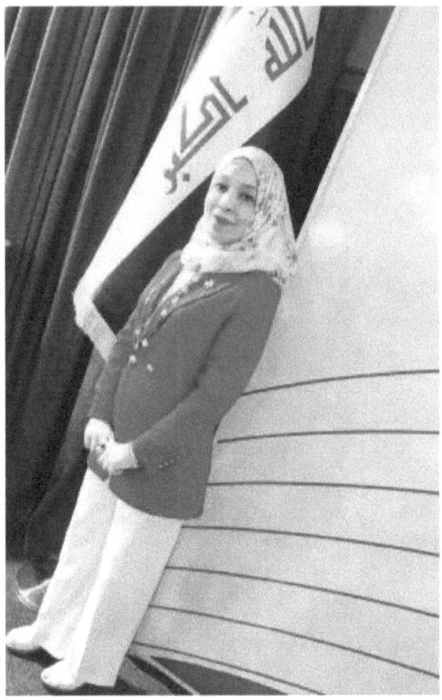

Assist. Prof. Dr. Zainab A.SHEHAB

Department of physiology, pharmacology and Biochemistry, College of veterinary medicine, University of Basrah, Iraq

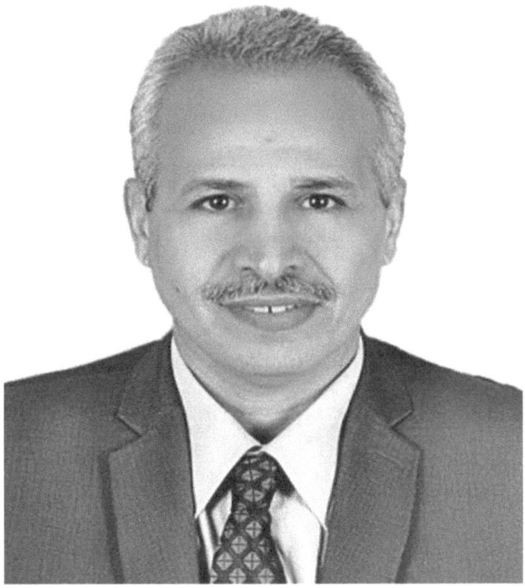

Prof. Dr. Mohamed Abdel-Raheem Ali Abdel-Raheem

Professor of Entomology (Biological Control)

Pests & Plant Protection Department

Agricultural and Biological Research Institute

National Research Centre.

Dr. Hind A. A. Alahmed

Department of physiology, pharmacology and Biochemistry, College of veterinary medicine, University of Basrah, Iraq

Content list

Introduction

While externally distinct, an elephant, a sunflower, and an amoeba share a common internal composition, consisting of the same fundamental building blocks. Whether it is the single cells found in basic organisms or the numerous cells that form the intricate structure of the human body, all living beings on Earth are ultimately composed of cells.

This concept, a fundamental aspect of biology, is a key principle of the cell theory. According to this theory, cells serve as the basic functional unit of living organisms and are all derived from pre-existing cells. Despite its significance in modern science, early researchers were unaware of the existence of cells.

The development of the microscope played a crucial role in unraveling the mysteries of the microscopic world. Renowned scientist Robert Hooke, eager to explore this realm, enhanced the design of the compound microscope in 1665. His innovative microscope, equipped with three lenses and a stage light, allowed for the illumination and magnification of specimens.

The technological advancements during Hooke's time allowed him to make a fascinating discovery when examining a piece of cork under a microscope. His detailed observations of this minuscule and previously unseen world were documented in his book called Micrographia. Upon closer inspection, Hooke observed that the cork appeared to consist of small pores, which he cleverly named "cells" due to their resemblance to cells found in a monastery.

In his writings in Micrographia, Hooke described the cells in cork as being perforated and porous, resembling a honeycomb but with irregular pores. These cells were the first microscopic structures he had ever observed, and perhaps the first ever seen by anyone, as he had not come across any references to them in any previous works or discussions.

Shortly after Robert Hooke's groundbreaking discovery, Dutch scientist Antonie van Leeuwenhoek made his own significant find by detecting minute organisms such as bacteria and protozoa. Van Leeuwenhoek's proficiency as a skilled microscope creator allowed him to refine the design of the simple microscope, incorporating a single lens that could magnify objects by two to three hundred times their original size. What Van Leeuwenhoek observed through these

Van Leeuwenhoek's curiosity continued to grow, leading him to become the first person to observe and document spermatozoa in 1677. He also examined the dental plaque in his teeth under the microscope, discovering tiny living creatures he described as "animalcules" in a letter to the Royal Society.

In the nineteenth century, biologists began to closely study animal and plant tissues, advancing cell theory. Although it was evident that plants consisted entirely of cells with cell walls, the absence of a cell wall in animal cells posed a challenge. Many scientists at the time believed that animals were composed of "globules."

German scientists Theodore Schwann and Mattias Schleiden conducted in-depth studies on animal and plant cells, respectively. They identified crucial distinctions between these two types of cells and proposed the concept that cells served as the fundamental building blocks of both plants and animals.

However, Schwann and Schleiden had misconceptions about the process of cell growth. Schleiden's belief was that cells originated as "seeds" from the nucleus and developed from there. Similarly, Schwann theorized that animal cells formed through a process of "crystallization" within the material between existing cells. Subsequently, further scientific exploration began to reveal the accurate understanding of cell development. A crucial addition to the cell theory was made by Rudolf Virchow in 1855, asserting that all cells originate from pre-existing cells.

Towards the end of the 19th century, the focus of research shifted towards cytogenetics, a field that aimed to establish connections between cell studies and genetics. During the 1880s, it was Walter Sutton and Theodor Boveri who highlighted the chromosome as a central element of heredity, thereby forever intertwining the studies of genetics and cytology. Additional breakthroughs in the understanding of the role of cells in heredity came from the work of James Watson and Francis Crick, who delved into the structure of DNA.

The impact of the discovery of the cell persisted in scientific advancements a century later, particularly with the identification of stem cells, which are undifferentiated cells yet to specialize into specific cell types. Embryonic stem cells were first derived from mice in the 1980s, and in 1998, James Thomson successfully isolated human embryonic stem cells and cultivated cell lines. His research findings were subsequently published in a notable article in the journal Science. Furthermore, it was revealed that adult tissues, predominantly skin cells, could be reprogrammed into stem cells and then differentiated into other specialized cell types, now referred to as induced pluripotent stem cells. Stem cells have now become integral in the treatment of various conditions such as Alzheimer's and heart disease.

The impact of the discovery of the cell in 1665 has surpassed even Hooke's wildest dreams. This groundbreaking revelation not only provides a profound insight into the fundamental components of all living organisms but has also paved the way for remarkable advancements in medical science and treatment. Modern scientists are currently engaged in the field of personalized medicine, utilizing stem cells derived from an individual's own cells to delve into the intricacies of various disease processes. All of these remarkable developments have emanated from a simple observation of a cell within a cork.

Regenerative medicine, a specialized branch of medical science, focuses on the innovation and implementation of techniques aimed at fostering the growth, repair, or replacement of damaged or unhealthy cells, organs, or tissues. In recent times, regenerative medicine has gained significant traction and attention. Stem cells, possessing the unique ability to self-renew and differentiate into specialized tissue cells, are integral to the advancements in this field.

Stem cell therapies are particularly important for addressing the challenges arise from the body's restricted capacity to repair and rejuvenate injured tissues and metabolic processes after experiencing acute or chronic damage. The origin of stem cell therapy can be traced back to 1991 when Caplan introduced the concept. Caplan theorized that the manipulation of stem cells in a controlled laboratory setting could lead to the significant development of specific tissues. Among the various types of stem cells, Mesenchymal stem cells (MSC) are particularly favored for therapeutic applications because of their straightforward isolation and cultivation processes, as well as the absence of ethical concerns surrounding their use among the various types of stem cells. Their ability to modulate the immune system is increasingly acknowledged in veterinary medicine.

The advancements in this specific field have primarily been propelled by the inadequacies of current treatment options for different medical ailments in a range of animal species. Mesenchymal stem cells offer a hopeful therapeutic solution for numerous animal illnesses, including orthopedic, orodental, and gastrointestinal disorders, as well as conditions impacting the liver, kidneys, heart, lungs, muscles, skin, olfactory senses, and reproductive system.

Despite progress in understanding the behavior and mechanisms of action of MSCs, there are lingering concerns regarding their adequacy for use in therapeutic settings.

Stem cells, by definition, are cells that have not yet differentiated and possess the ability to both self-renew and develop into various specialized cell types. These cells are categorized based on their origin as embryonic, adult, or induced pluripotent stem cells. Furthermore, depending on their stage in the realm of cell development and specialization, cells can be categorized as totipotent, pluripotent, or multipotent based on their level of differentiation. [1- 4].

Totipotent stem cells are characterized by their ability to differentiate into any type of cell in the human body, predominantly located during the initial phases of embryo growth, notably in the morula stage preceding gastrulation. These cells possess the extraordinary capability to develop into a wide array of embryonic and extra-embryonic tissues. As cell division progresses in the early stages of embryo development, they ultimately form the blastocyst, in which pluripotent embryonic stem cells (ESC) are located within the inner cell mass. ESC have the capacity to differentiate into any type of tissue cell within the body, excluding extra-embryonic tissues and germ cells. As development progresses, pluripotent ESC gradually lose their pluripotency and transition to a multipotent state. This stage is marked by the ability of cells to differentiate into a limited range of specific cell types, typically based on their original germ layer lineage.[2, 5, 6]

The initial derivation of human embryonic stem cells was officially documented in 1998, prompting a surge in research exploring gene activity and roles during embryonic growth and cell specialization processes. Efforts were also made to pinpoint genes suitable for new pharmaceuticals that could be beneficial in tissue rejuvenation treatments. Nevertheless, the vast therapeutic potential of human embryonic stem cells clashed with moral, ethical, and cultural concerns due to the necessity of using human embryos for their collection [7].

Exploration of alternative reservoirs of stem cells was deemed necessary in order to progress the research and implementation of stem cell-based therapies. A groundbreaking technique was unveiled by Takahashi and Yamanaka in 2006, which involved the reprogramming of adult mouse fibroblasts into pluripotent stem cells through the introduction of four distinct genes - OCT4, c-Myc, SOX2, and KLF4 - via retroviral vectors. These cells were referred to as induced pluripotent stem cells (IPSC) and exhibited similarities to embryonic stem cells in terms of appearance, growth characteristics, and the presence of embryonic stem cell markers. [8]

Although the creation of IPSC marked a significant advancement in stem cell therapy, concerns arose regarding the use of retroviral transductions, which could lead to chromosomal irregularities and an elevated risk of tumor formation, thereby casting doubt on the medicine purposes.[3]

An alternative to embryonic stem cells is the presence of stem cells in adult organisms. Cells are classified as multipotent due to their ability to develop into specific types of cells within the body [9].

Hematopoietic stem cells (HSCs) possess the ability to differentiate into a variety of cells within the immune system, as well as erythrocytes and platelets. Meanwhile, Mesenchymal stem cells (MSCs) have the capacity to differentiate into various types of cells found in bone, cartilage, ligaments, tendons, adipose tissue, skin, muscle, and connective tissue, these components are present.

MSCs are naturally mobilized within the body to regenerate and replace damaged or dying tissue cells. The initial discovery of adult multipotent cells/MSCs can be dated back to 1968, when a group of osteogenic cells displaying a fibroblast-like morphology were identified in bone marrow. Early studies exhibited the potential of multipotent stem cells to differentiate transformed into cells such as osteoblasts, chondroblasts, and adipocytes. [10].

It is widely believed that mesenchymal stem cells exhibit their therapeutic effectiveness through differentiation into various tissue-specific cells. Recent studies have cast doubt on this notion, suggesting that the predominant source of MSC's regenerative capabilities lies in their immunomodulatory and tissue repair functions.

It is theorized that the perivascular positioning of MSCs in different tissues is crucial in allowing them to identify and react to local or remote tissue damage by migrating specifically site of injury and contributing to process. [11-13].

In his work, Caplan suggested a change in terminology from "mesenchymal stem cells" to "medicinal signaling cell" (MSC) [14].

Among various types of stem cells, MSCs are considered the most promising for stem cell therapy due to their ease of harvest, isolation, high yield, and ethical considerations. To address confusion in the field, the committee dedicated to the investigation of Mesenchymal and Tissue Stem Cells within the International Society for Cellular Therapy (ISCT) is being conducted. established standards for defining human MSCs in research and studies [15].

This entails that MSCs should adhere to plastic under standard culture conditions, express specific markers, and exhibit differentiation capacity into specific cell types under controlled laboratory conditions.[16-20]

Thus far, Mesenchymal Stem Cells (MSCs) have been successfully obtained from a variety of tissues, each possessing distinct properties based on their origin. This differentiation should be taken into account when selecting the most effective stem cell therapy for tissue regeneration. [21- 27] Among the most common companion animals treated in veterinary practice, including dogs, horses, and cats, MSCs have been harvested from bone marrow, adipose tissue, synovium, synovial fluid, synovial membrane, infrapatellar fat pad, umbilical cord, umbilical cord blood, Wharton's Jelly, muscle and periosteum, gingiva and periodontal ligament, peripheral blood, endometrium, and placenta.[28-31]

MSCs were isolated from various tissues in mice including Various organs in the body such as the brain, spleen, liver, kidney, lung, muscle, thymus, and pancreas serve as vital reservoirs of Mesenchymal Stem Cells (MSC) that are harnessed for stem cell treatments. The primary sources of MSC commonly utilized in these therapies include bone marrow and adipose tissue, primarily due to their abundance in the body. Adipose tissue, in particular, is favored for its straightforward collection process. Although MSCs derived from bone marrow and adipose tissue exhibit similar characteristics, there are variances in their proliferative and differentiation capabilities, as well as their secretion profiles. [32-37]

Studies have indicated that canine adipose tissue derived MSCs have a higher proliferation rate than bone marrow derived MSCs, while the latter exhibit An increased secretion of soluble factors and exosomes is observed in Canine ADMSCs. Furthermore, Canine ADMSCs exhibit superior capabilities in chondrogenesis and osteogenesis when compared to BMMSCs. Conversely, in equine subjects, BMMSCs demonstrate a greater potential for both chondrogenesis and osteogenesis than ADMSCs. [38-43].

Equine bone marrow-derived mesenchymal stem cells appear to exhibit a greater ability to migrate compared to adipose tissue-derived MSCs. Synovium-derived MSCs could also be Adipose-derived stem cells are considered a promising reservoir of cells with significant potential for cartilage regeneration. Research has shown these cells to possess a greater capacity for rapid proliferation compared to other types of stem cells in horses and exhibit superior abilities in cartilage formation when compared to cells derived from adipose tissue and bone marrow in canines. Therefore, careful consideration of the specific location from which adipose tissue is obtained is crucial when choosing it as a source of mesenchymal stem cells. [44, 45]

Studies have demonstrated that adipose-derived mesenchymal stem cells (ADMSCs) from subcutaneous fat exhibit a heightened capacity for cell proliferation compared to those derived from visceral fat depots. Furthermore, research suggests that subcutaneous ADMSCs retain their ability to differentiate into multiple cell types for a longer period in culture and display superior potential for bone formation. In addition, it has been observed that visceral adipose tissue yields a greater quantity of mesenchymal stem cells (MSCs) compared to subcutaneous adipose tissue. [46]

Given that variations in stem cell characteristics may impact the outcomes of stem cell therapy, it is imperative to conduct further investigation into these differences. Currently, there is a lack of definitive evidence supporting a preferred tissue source for MSCs, Variations in donor species, age, and health conditions in various studies contribute to the complexity of research outcomes. The lack of standardized procedures for isolating, culturing, and characterizing animal MSCs presents difficulties in comparing results across studies. Additionally, the diverse range of tissue sources further complicates the analysis complicates the establishment of MSC-defining criteria.

At present, there are no universally accepted criteria for identifying MSCs in animals, unlike the criteria established for human MSCs. While all animal MSCs exhibit adherence to plastic and differentiation potential, not all share the same set of surface antigens commonly associated with human MSCs. Most non-human MSCs express CD29 and CD44, but the presence of CD73, CD90, and CD105 varies depending on the species and strain. [47].

According to the relationship between the donor and recipient, stem cells can be categorized as autologous, allogeneic, or xenogeneic. Autologous stem cells are obtained and transferred within the same individual, allogeneic stem cells are collected from a donor and utilized in a recipient of the same species, and xenogeneic stem cells are transplanted between different species. [48].

When selecting the most suitable cells for specific stem cell therapy, the decision between autologous and allogeneic sources can present difficulties. It is important to weigh the advantages and disadvantages of each option. Isolating and expanding autologous stem cells is a time-consuming and costly process. Furthermore, the efficacy of autologous mesenchymal stem cells can be influenced by the age of the patient as well as any preexisting medical conditions. This has led to an increasing demand for allogeneic stem cell products sourced from young and healthy donors [49-54].

Allogeneic stem cell therapy raises a significant issue concerning the potential interaction between MHC I surface proteins on allogeneic MSCs and recipient CD8+ T cells, which could induce direct cell death against the foreign cells. Furthermore, the identification of MHC II molecules by recipient CD4+ T cells may result in cytotoxic or humoral immune responses. Additionally, MHC molecules could be indirectly detected by antigen presenting cells, potentially stimulating the production of alloantibodies in B cells. [55].

Although initial studies have shown promising results in terms of the safety of allogeneic mesenchymal stem cells (MSC), subsequent research conducted both in vitro and in vivo, including studies in rodents, horses, and dogs, have demonstrated immunogenic responses elicited by allogeneic MSC[56- 61. These findings have raised concerns regarding the perceived immunoprivileged nature of these cells. In specific studies conducted [62- 64]local side effects were observed following repeated administration of allogeneic cells, with adverse reactions believed to be primarily attributed to immune recognition by the recipient after subsequent exposure. [65].

For example, Menard et al. [66] Studies have demonstrated that Adipose-Derived Mesenchymal Stem Cells (ADMSCs) exhibit an enhanced ability to regulate immune cells and their characteristics align with a lower level of immunogenicity when compared to Bone Marrow-Derived Mesenchymal Stem Cells (BMMSCs).

Despite the promising findings from various studies supporting the use of allogeneic MSCs, there have been reports indicating that the immunosuppressive nature of MSCs does not completely eliminate their potential for immunogenicity. Further investigations are necessary to identify possible mechanisms for controlling Major Histocompatibility Complex.

Initially believed to act as a reservoir for cells with the capacity to differentiate and regenerate damaged tissues, it is now evident that the therapeutic benefits of MSCs predominantly derive from their immunomodulatory functions, which are executed through their interactions with immune system cells.

The intricate immunomodulatory capabilities of MSCs encompass their paracrine functioning, the release of extracellular vesicles (ECV), immunomodulation via apoptosis, and the transmission of membrane vesicles and organelles via mitochondria. Growing evidence indicates that the main mode of action of MSCs is through paracrine signaling, triggering alterations in the behavior of immune cells like monocytes/macrophages, dendritic cells, T-cells, B-cells, and natural killer cells. [66- 71].

Numerous elements have been identified as contributors to the immunomodulatory impacts of Mesenchymal Stem Cells. Some well-known mediators include Factors such as transforming growth factor-beta (TGF-β), indoleamine-2,3-dioxygenase (IDO), prostaglandin E2 (PGE2), interleukin 10 (IL-10), and tumor necrosis factor-stimulated gene-6 play a significant role in the process of transformation. [72-74]

TGF-β plays a crucial role in a variety of biological processes including cell proliferation, embryonic development, wound healing, and angiogenesis. It influences the migration, adhesion, and maturation of Mesenchymal Stem Cells (MSCs). In addition, research has demonstrated that TGF-β is involved in promoting a transition from an inflammatory (M1) to an anti-inflammatory/regulatory (M2) state in macrophages, which in turn contributes significantly to the development of regulatory T-cells (Tregs). [75–79].

IDO, an enzyme involved in metabolism, is a soluble factor that is released by mesenchymal stem cells in the presence of inflammation. IDO is responsible for regulating the cell cycle of T and B cells, suppressing T-cell growth, promoting the generation of regulatory T cells, inhibiting B cells and NK cells, and influencing the differentiation of M2 macrophages.[80-83] Additionally, PGE2, a primary prostaglandin, Plays a significant part in modulating the production of chemokines, inhibiting the influx of inflammatory cells, and facilitating the formation of regulatory cells. [84].

IL-10 is essential for facilitating NK-cell suppression and shaping the development of macrophages into the M2 phenotype. Recent research has demonstrated its role in facilitating the removal of apoptotic cells by MSC. Known for its anti-inflammatory qualities, this cytokine effectively regulates both Th1 and Th2 responses and modulates the activities of macrophages and dendritic cells. Furthermore, IL-10 hinders the proliferation of T-cells while enhancing the generation of Tregs. [85- 91].

TSG-6 is a protein linked to inflammation that possesses anti-inflammatory and protective attributes. MSCs consistently produce TSG-6, influencing various aspects of their functionality such as morphology, extracellular vesicle size, growth rate, potential for differentiation, viability, and capacity for forming colonies, thus playing a critical role in preserving their stem cell characteristics. Research has demonstrated that TSG-6 prompts the transition from an M1 to an M2 phenotype and enhances the presence of Tregs, ultimately alleviating symptoms associated with inflammatory disorders in experimental disease models [92–95].

MSCs have the ability to influence the progression and outcomes of a specific disease by modulating an individual's immune response through their paracrine effects. The paracrine activity of MSCs extends beyond the release of soluble substances is accompanied by the ability to transport different molecules through extracellular vesicles (ECV). [96-98] Extracellular vesicles (ECVs) are phospholipid bilayer-bound particles that are formed from the plasma membrane via internal or external budding mechanisms. These vesicles encapsulate various cargo such as miRNA, mRNA, proteins, and mitochondria within their membrane, enabling them to traverse long distances in the body efficiently. Among the different categories of ECVs are exosomes, which are small vesicles derived from endocytosis and typically range in size from 30 to 150 nm. Microvesicles, on the other hand, originate from cellular outward budding processes and vary in size 100 to 1000 nm, and apoptotic bodies released during membrane blebbing of apoptotic cells and measuring from 50 nm to 5 μm [99].

MSCs have demonstrated the ability to release exosomes along with a minimum of three other equivalently sized extracellular vesicle types. [100].

In terms of the mechanisms of action of extracellular vesicles (ECVs), they appear to parallel those of mesenchymal stem cells (MSCs) themselves. A study conducted [101, 102] highlighted that ECVs can stimulate M2 macrophages in a similar manner to MSCs by activating prostaglandin E2 (PGE2). Additionally, recent research findings indicate that ECVs can inhibit T-cells through signaling pathways involving transforming growth factor-beta (TGF-β) and adenosine. The main responsibility for promoting regulatory T cells (Tregs) was credited to tumor necrosis factor-inducible gene 6 protein (TSG-6) found in ECVs derived from adipose tissue-derived MSCs in a study focusing on therapeutic treatment for induced colitis in mice. Moreover, it was demonstrated that ECVs had the capacity to enhance the expression of interleukin 10 (IL-10) in a murine sepsis model when introduced. [103].

In animal models such as pigs, mice, and rats, studies have shown that extracellular vesicles derived from mesenchymal stem cells have demonstrated therapeutic benefits in respiratory, renal, and liver diseases, as well as in the management of conditions such as osteoarthritis, spinal cord injury, cerebral ischemia, and myocardial infarction. [104-11] Additionally, these extracellular vesicles have shown promising results in dogs and horses.

Utilizing microvesicles derived from adipose-derived mesenchymal stem cells resulted in enhanced angiogenesis and increased elasticity in a damaged tendon of a stallion. Additionally, in canines, extracellular vesicles have been shown to promote vascularization, stimulate collagen production, and expedite the healing of skin wounds more effectively than the parent cells themselves. [112].

Extracellular vesicles (EVs) offer the opportunity to harness the therapeutic benefits of mesenchymal stem cell (MSC) effects without the risk of adverse reactions associated with direct MSC administration, such as immune rejection and pulmonary embolism. However, it is acknowledged that cellular interactions play a crucial role in certain immunomodulatory functions attributed to MSCs. [68, 70, 113].

Upon administration through the vein, heat-treated MSCs that lack secreted proteins but have intact cell membrane were observed to have a comparable effect on monocyte activity as regular cells. This resulted in an increase in IL-10 levels and a decrease in IFN-γ levels.

These findings imply that the immune response following MSC administration may not rely on their active immunomodulatory capabilities. It appears that mere interaction with MSCs is adequate to induce certain immunomodulatory responses.[114]

The main challenge in the study of extracellular vesicles (ECVs) is the lack of standardized protocols for isolating and purifying these vesicles. Various methods commonly used for isolating exosomes include Techniques such as ultracentrifugation, ultrafiltration, tangential flow filtration, precipitation, size exclusion chromatography, and immunoaffinity-based methods are commonly utilized for the isolation of exosomes. Key biomarkers for exosomes include caveolins, clathrins, transferrin receptors, tetraspanins (CD81, CD63, CD9), Alix, and TSG101, are linked to endocytosis. Variations in ligands and cargo among different ECV types suggest distinct functions for each type. The lack of standardized isolation methods hinders the ability to differentiate exosomes from similarly sized ECVs. Additionally, there is currently no universally accepted measure of ECV purity, leading to inconsistencies in the literature regarding their characterization [115- 117].

The Association for Extracellular Vesicles on a global scale recommends that researchers use the term extracellular vesicle instead of a specific subtype, unless specifically defined. It is recommended to provide comprehensive explanations of isolation and preparation methods to facilitate reproducibility. Emphasizing the necessity of confirming extracellular vesicle function involves demonstrating that their impact occurs in the absence of direct cell-to-cell communication and cannot be replicated with soluble factors not linked to extracellular vesicles. [118].

Apoptosis can greatly influence the immunomodulatory functions of MSCs. Efferocytosis, the phagocytic removal of dying cells, not only aids in resolving inflammation and regenerating furthermore, it plays a dual role in not only maintaining the integrity of the tissue but also aiding in the regulation of adaptive and immune responses within inflamed tissues. Luk et al. conducted a study indicating that heat-inactivated MSCs modulated monocyte function similarly to control cells, leading to increased levels of IL-10 and decreased levels of IFN-γ.

The immune response triggered by the administration of MSCs is the effectiveness of the treatment does not rely exclusively on the active immunomodulatory characteristics of the cells, but is also impacted by the presence of other cell types. that are activated in response to the presence of MSCs. Recent studies have indicated that cells of the innate immune system play a crucial role in mediating the effects of MSCs. Galleu et al. recently demonstrated through their research that MSCs undergo apoptosis when exposed to cytotoxic cells such as CD56+ NK cells and CD8+ T-cells post intravenous infusion. This apoptosis of MSCs induced by cytotoxic cells does not rely on MHC and necessitates direct interaction between MSCs and cytotoxic cells. [119]

Following apoptosis, mesenchymal stem cells (MSCs) are engulfed by macrophages, which subsequently release immunosuppressive activity through the production of IDO. Studies by Cheung et al. have demonstrated a similar process, wherein monocytes that have phagocytosed apoptotic MSCs enhance the suppression of T-cell growth through the production of prostaglandin E2. The mechanism of immunosuppression derived from apoptosis could potentially serve as a predictive factor in clinical treatments, particularly for patients exhibiting elevated cytotoxicity who may show greater responsiveness to MSC therapy [120, 121].

Mesenchymal Stem Cells (MSCs) were delivered intravenously to mice, they were quickly engulfed by monocytes and neutrophils in the lungs. This phagocytosis of MSCs leads to the induction of a regulatory phenotype in monocytes and encourages their polarization, consequently impacting the adaptive immune system by activating T-reg cells. [122]

Additionally, mitochondrial transfer has been proposed as an additional mechanism by which MSCs exert their effects. In addition to transferring molecules via Extracellular Vesicles (ECVs), MSCs may also transfer organelles through tunneling nanotubes between cells. The initial documented case of mitochondrial transfer from MSCs to somatic cells took place in 2006. This seminal study demonstrated that the active transfer of mitochondria from adult stem cells to somatic cells could potentially restore aerobic respiration in mammalian cells with impaired mitochondria. [123]

It was observed that human bone marrow-derived mesenchymal stem cells (BMMSC) were able to transfer their mitochondria to alveolar macrophages through tunneling nanotubes. This transfer resulted in an increased phagocytic activity of the macrophages and enhanced antimicrobial effects of the MSCs.[124]

Given the association of mitochondrial transfer with various physiological and pathological processes, this mechanism holds potential for the treatment of a wide range of pathological conditions.[125]

In addition to their intricate immunomodulatory functions, a major advantage of mesenchymal stem cell (MSC)-based therapies lies in their capacity to home in on damaged tissue. The homing of MSCs is closely linked to chemical factors such as chemokines, cytokines, and growth factors. Stromal cell-derived factor 1 (SDF-1) is a key chemical factor that plays a crucial role in promoting the migration of MSCs. [126].

In non-activated mesenchymal stem cells (MSCs), the expression of CXCR4 is constrained on the cellular membrane while being intensified intracellularly. Upon activation, MSCs undergo a rapid relocation of CXCR4 receptors to the cell surface, enabling them to efficiently respond to signals triggering cell migration. [127- 129]

Various chemokine receptors, such as CCR6, CCR9, CXCR3, and CXCR6, have been recognized on the membranes of MSCs, in addition to CXCR4, and are essential for the migration of MSCs. [130- 134] Osteopontin (OPN), a molecule that is elevated in damaged tissues and inflammation, functions to attract mesenchymal stem cells (MSCs) in response to osteopontin stimulation, mesenchymal stem cells are attracted to areas of injury by interacting with integrin β1 receptors. The recruitment of MSCs is influenced by a variety of growth factors, such as fibroblast growth factor, vascular endothelial growth factor, hepatocyte growth factor, insulin-like growth factor-1, and TGF-β1. Additionally, mechanical factors like mechanical strain, shear stress, matrix rigidity, and microgravity are pivotal in the recruitment process of MSCs. [135].

In the realm of stem cell therapies, the local transplantation of MSC is considered an optimal approach for cell administration. Nevertheless, there are scenarios [136]

As a result, systemic applications, particularly through the intravenous route which is less invasive, are often the preferred method. The process of MSC homing following intravenous administration encounters several challenges. [137].

Furthermore, following intravenous transplantation, mesenchymal stem cells (MSCs) are frequently sequestered and subsequently eliminated from the pulmonary system. [138] MSCs are characterized by a relatively large size, averaging 30 μm in suspension, which contrasts with the average diameter of pulmonary capillaries at only 14 μm, leading to their mechanical entrapment in the lungs. Apart from their size, the molecular interactions between MSCs and the pulmonary endothelium may also contribute to their accumulation in this organ. Research conducted by Wang and colleagues highlighted the crucial role of integrins in the entrapment of MSCs within lung tissue. By blocking integrins, researchers observed a significant reduction in a mouse model, there was observed retention of MSCs in the lungs, an elevation in the concentration [139-143]

Observations from the monitoring of MSCs post systemic infusion revealed that these cells have a short lifespan, often disappearing within 24 hours. However, the extended advantages of MSCs seem to conflict with their temporary presence. It is noteworthy that the healing influence of MSCs may not be contingent on their viability, as demonstrated by the study conducted by de Witte and colleagues. Despite the short survival time and entrapment in the lungs following intravenous administration, MSCs exert a lasting inducing programmed cell death known as apoptosis and engulfment by immune cells. [144]

In order to prevent complications associated with intravenous administration, alternative routes of delivery have been explored, including intra-arterial (IA) and intraperitoneal (IP) routes. IA administration has the potential to decrease the build-up of mesenchymal stem cells (MSC) in filtering organs, making it a viable option for treating ischemic injuries. The injection of MSC via the IA route could lead to more even distribution of cells throughout the body. A research study conducted on a healthy porcine model revealed that the intravascular administration of MSCs through the femoral artery resulted in a higher distribution of MSCs in different organs, with a notable concentration [98].

The occurrence of thrombosis was notably absent in instances where intra-arterial injection was administered without the application of a tourniquet, suggesting that blood stasis, rather than the application of MSCs, may be the primary factor contributing to thrombosis. [145- 147].

In the same manner, the feasibility of intrarterial (IA) injection of mesenchymal stem cells (MSC) was demonstrated by researchers injecting allogeneic equine bone marrow-derived MSC [148, 149]

Although intraperitoneal (IP) administration of MSCs is not commonly practiced, it offers the potential to target intraabdominal regions and has shown to be relatively safe in feline subjects. [150].

The effectiveness of MSCs delivered intraperitoneally has been shown in rat studies for treating bladder detrusor dysfunction and in mouse models for inflammatory bowel disease. [151] Moreover, this method of delivery was employed in an initial investigation, overseen by the FDA, to infuse Neo-islets - a mixture of ADMSCs and pancreatic islet cells - into diabetic pet dogs reliant on insulin. The Neo-islets were observed to successfully integrate, differentiate, and generate insulin without provoking any immune response. [152].

Many patients undergoing treatment with MSCs are afflicted with acute or chronic inflammatory conditions, suggesting that an inflammatory milieu may prevail in vivo during MSC administration. By pre-treating MSCs with IFN-γ, the intention is to simulate the in vivo environment in which these cells will operate. It has been theorized that under inflammatory circumstances, the interaction between MSCs and B-cells could be intensified.

Mesenchymal stem cells (MSCs) cultured in an inflamed environment significantly impeded the proliferation of B-cells and the production of IgG by activating indoleamine-2,3-dioxygenase [102]

Other research has highlighted potential drawbacks of conditioning MSCs with pro-inflammatory cytokines. For example, pretreatment with IFN-gamma increased the immunogenicity of MSCs by upregulating the expression of MHC and MHC II. [153–156].

Treatment with both IFN-γ and TNF-α was demonstrated to induce apoptosis in murine MSCs. This apoptotic response was triggered by the upregulation of inducible nitric oxide synthase (iNOS) and the subsequent production of nitric oxide - both critical for the initiation of apoptosis. In order to minimize the potential negative consequences of preconditioning with IFN-γ while simultaneously enhancing their immunosuppressive properties, a suggested alternative is to pretreat MSCs with IL-17A. [156, 157].

Brandt et al. [158] conducted a study which revealed that equine ADMSCs face challenges when exposed to an inflammatory environment. The presence of high levels of proinflammatory cytokines such as TNF-α and IL-1β, as well as leukocytes, led to an increase in the proliferation potential and osteogenic differentiation of ADMSCs. The mixed findings from various research studies on pre-conditioning MSCs with proinflammatory cytokines indicate that although there may be some potential benefits from such treatments, they should be approached with caution. Further investigation is required to fully understand the potential positive impacts of such pre-conditioning methods.

The utilization of mesenchymal stem cells in the field of Veterinary Medicine for therapeutic purposes

To this point in time, stem cells have primarily been utilized in an experimental capacity for the treatment of a range of diseases across various animal species.

Initially, regenerative veterinary medicine emphasized orthopedic conditions, but there has been a notable shift towards exploring treatments for orodental ailments. Stem cell therapies have been predominantly employed in dogs and horses for a multitude of organ system disorders, as well as in cats for conditions affecting the kidneys, respiratory system, and inflammatory responses.

Conditions affecting the musculoskeletal system

Tendon and ligament disorders

Injuries to tendons and ligaments resulting from trauma and stress often heal through the formation of scar tissue that does not possess the same functionality as healthy tissue.

Consequently, this compromises the individual's ability to move effectively and increases the risk of re-injury. [159, 160].

The optimal treatment strategy should prioritize the restoration of the tissue's natural form and function. Traditional methods for addressing tendon injuries in horses encompass measures such as cooling, wrapping, and a closely supervised rehabilitation regimen incorporating controlled physical activity. Pharmaceutical treatments may consist of the use of systemic or localized corticosteroids, in addition to other anti-inflammatory drugs.

In some cases, surgical intervention may be necessary. [161- 164]. The traditional methods employed do not facilitate full tissue recovery, resulting in a high likelihood of reinjury. As a consequence, animals frequently struggle to regain their preinjury level of performance [162].

An ideal treatment approach should focus on restoring Mesenchymal stem cell (MSC) therapy has become a promising alternative to traditional approaches in enhancing tissue regeneration by targeting the normal tendon matrix. [165]

Research suggests that utilizing MSC derived from the same tissue requiring treatment is the most optimal source for stem cell therapy. [166, 167]

Tendon-derived stem cells are widely regarded as the optimal choice for treating tendinopathies, despite the intricate nature of extracting stem cells from tendon tissue and the absence of a universally accepted method for inducing tendon formation. Consequently, alternative sources such as adipose tissue and bone marrow have been explored for regenerating tendons. In 2003, the first recorded instance of autologous bone marrow-derived mesenchymal stem cell (BMMSC) implantation in a horse's superficial digital flexor tendon took place. [168].

After administering cells to 11 racehorses with superficial digital flexor tendon lesions, a notable improvement in clinical symptoms was noticed. Another study involving 141 racehorses with naturally occurring superficial digital flexor tendon injuries found that the use of autologous cells resulted in promising outcomes.

Note: The provided text is incomplete BMMSCs for intralesional injections resulted in less than 28% reinjury rate in all horses over a two-year period. [169] This result signified a notable reduction in re-injury rates when compared to a prior study that focused on treating horses [170].

Smith et al. [171] demonstrated that autologous Bone Marrow Mesenchymal Stem Cell (BMMSC) treatment in cases of tendinopathies leads to the development of a tissue composition [173- 177].

Several research studies have demonstrated the beneficial effects of utilizing MSCs in this particular medical condition. The findings indicate that administering a single intra-articular injection of allogeneic BMMSCs could potentially be a more effective treatment option for reducing post-operative lameness and pain compared to a one-month course of oral NSAIDs in dogs undergoing TPLO surgery. [178- 180].

A retrospective study yielded encouraging outcomes for cases of partial tears in the stifle joint without joint destabilization, where surgery may not be the preferred course of action. The study showed that utilizing autologous bone marrow-derived mesenchymal stem cells (BMMSC) in conjunction with platelet-rich plasma (PRP) effectively halted the advancement of degenerative alterations in the joint and prevented contralateral ligament rupture in dogs. [181].

Conditions affecting the joints

Due to its low cellularity and lack of blood vessels, cartilage tissue has a restricted ability to heal itself. In horses, this limitation is compounded by the substantial forces and mechanical stress endured by the articular surfaces during performance. Joint diseases, particularly osteoarthritis, are a leading cause of chronic lameness and premature retirement among equine athletes. Traditional approaches to treating musculoskeletal injuries [182- 186].

After the treatment period, it was observed that there was no presence of lameness in the horses that received treatment for 180 days, in contrast to the control group which did not receive treatment. This was confirmed by scintigraphy which revealed that there was no inflammation in the tarsal joints of the treated horses, while inflammation continued to be present in the control group.

MSC therapy also shows promise in cases of meniscal damage in horses, with those receiving intra-articular autologous BMMSC treatment demonstrating a higher rate of return to work compared to those treated solely with arthroscopy. [187].

In a particular study involving 80 horses suffering from osteoarthritis, treatment with allogeneic ADMSC resulted in a notable decrease in lameness over a 90-day period. This indicates the advantageous impact of allogeneic cells. Likewise. [65, 66]

Singular administration of allogeneic MSCs has also been associated with inducing mild to moderate localized inflammatory reactions. Various studies with canines have demonstrated that the introduction of MSCs into arthritic joints can alleviate discomfort and improve functional capacities in the animals. [188]

Dogs suffering from stifle osteoarthritis exhibited a noticeable reduction in lameness, supported by the considerably slower progression of osteoarthritis in joints treated with autologous ADMSCs as opposed to those given a placebo [189-194].

During a study involving dogs with osteoarthritis who were treated with allogeneic umbilical cord-derived MSCs, positive outcomes were observed, including the generation of new cartilage and decreased joint fluid, decreased inflammation, and improved tissue healing compared to the untreated control group. Research findings have indicated that repeated allogeneic MSC treatment in horses is safe, yielding only mild and transient inflammatory responses without any negative effects even two years post-injection. Additionally, the efficacy of MSC therapy for osteoarthritis in dogs, whether using the animal's own cells or donor cells [191, 195, 196].

Studies indicate that Mesenchymal Stem Cell (MSC) therapy has demonstrated superior efficacy compared to Platelet-Rich Plasma (PRP) therapy in the treatment of osteoarthritis in dogs. MSC therapy has exhibited notable advantages in addressing musculoskeletal ailments in horses, particularly in cases of tendon injuries, bone spavin, and meniscal damage, as well as in dogs suffering from osteoarthritis. [197]

The favorable outcomes of MSC therapies have led to a reduction in the necessity for prolonged administration of anti-inflammatory drugs with their associated harmful side effects. Nevertheless, further research is essential to enhance our understanding of the mechanisms of action of MSCs, including allogeneic MSCs, as some studies have not consistently reported positive outcomes regarding their safety in therapeutic applications.

MSC derived extracellular vesicles show potential as a viable substitute for allogeneic MSC therapy due to their ability to replicate many of the biological functions of MSCs. The efficacy of ECV therapy has been demonstrated in a study involving the treatment [111].

Afflictions affecting the mouth and teeth

Oral discomfort and problems with chewing can significantly impact the well-being of animals. Numerous oral conditions can also lead to broader health concerns. Conditions like tooth decay, gum disease, tooth loss, oral sores, throat cancer, and dental injuries are prevalent public health issues globally. The use of stem cells in regenerative therapy has emerged as a promising approach to healing oral and dental tissues.[198]

Research is concentrated on examining the immunomodulatory impacts of mesenchymal stem cells (MSCs) with the aim of stimulating the regeneration of oral tissues. Additionally, there is interest in investigating the capability of MSCs to improve the longevity of dental implants and rectify bone deficiencies in the jaw. Scholars are delving into the healing properties of stem cells harvested from local oral sources, such as dental pulp stem cells (DPSC) and periodontal ligament stem cells (PDLSC), in the treatment of oral and dental ailments. [199-204]

Moreover, allogeneic ADMSCs have displayed the capacity to promote the regeneration of periodontal tissues in a mini pig model of periodontal defects.

In relation to the regeneration of dental pulp, studies have shown that both autologous and allogeneic stem cells derived from dental pulp, as well as autologous bone marrow-derived mesenchymal stem cells (BMMSCs), have displayed effectiveness in restoring dental pulp in canine subjects.

While the findings suggest promise for regenerating orodental tissues, some research has indicated that there are limited benefits connected to the use of stem cells in addressing dental problems like issues related to dental implants. [205-209].

Research conducted on animal subjects serves as a fundamental framework and a source of guidance for utilizing stem cells and tissue engineering to improve the regeneration of oral and dental tissues.

However, further comprehensive research is required to confirm the efficacy and feasibility of stem cell therapies for orodental disorders in real patients afflicted with naturally occurring ailments.

Cats experiencing FCGS typically exhibit symptoms such as loss of appetite, oral discomfort, weight loss, excessive drooling, bad breath, and neglect of grooming. Common treatment measures encompass the use of drugs like corticosteroids, cyclosporin, and tooth extraction procedures, all of which have varying rates of success and potential adverse effects. [210- 214].

Arzi and his team demonstrated in their study that the intravenous administration of autologous adipose-derived mesenchymal stem cells (ADMSC) led to complete clinical and histological improvement or reduction in disease severity in a majority of feline subjects. Additionally, the study highlighted the immunomodulatory effects of MSCs by restoring balance to immune cell subsets, serum protein levels, and cytokine levels.[215]

Moreover, the study suggested that the lack of CD8lo cells could potentially function as a biomarker for forecasting the effectiveness of MSC therapy.

It is worth noting that allogeneic ADMSCs exhibited lower clinical effectiveness compared to autologous MSCs in treating feline chronic gingivostomatitis (FCGS).

In a separate finding, the study revealed that 70% of cats with FCGS demonstrated a clinical, histological, and systemic response following intravenous administration of allogeneic ADMSCs. [217].

Diseases of the gastrointestinal system

Inflammatory bowel disease, known as IBD, is a long-term autoimmune disorder marked by a persistent hypersensitivity response in the intestinal mucosa with an unidentified cause. There are certain dogs that do not have a positive reaction to the customary lifelong therapies utilizing cyclosporine or steroids. After receiving a singular intravenous infusion of allogeneic ADMSCs, showing a significant increase in albumin, cobalamin, and folate levels in their blood. [218, 219].

In felines experiencing chronic vomiting and diarrhea, inflammatory bowel disease (IBD) is a frequent occurrence. A study involving a placebo-controlled group indicated that cats diagnosed with IBD experienced notable amelioration or complete eradication of clinical manifestations when administered allogeneic ADMSC, according to the reports of their caregivers. Conversely, cats in the placebo cohort either displayed no alteration in their condition or a deterioration in symptoms. [220]

Given their immunomodulatory and anti-inflammatory properties, mesenchymal stem cells (MSCs) appear to offer a promising alternative for treating IBD in dogs and cats.

Liver ailments

Numerous studies have specifically examined the use of stem cell therapy in the treatment of liver disease in dogs. Examined the effects of intravenously introducing autologous adipose-derived mesenchymal stem cells (ADMSC) to dogs with experimentally-induced acute hepatic injury. The study's results indicated that ADMSC successfully traveled to the liver, leading to a decrease in liver enzyme levels in the blood and restoration of liver tissue structure after treatment, suggesting promising potential for mesenchymal stem cells (MSC) in managing liver diseases in companion animals. Furthermore, MSC were utilized in a separate study involving a canine model with liver cirrhosis. In this research, intravenous administration of autologous bone marrow-derived mesenchymal stem cells (BMMSC) led to a notable reduction in liver fibrosis area and enhancement in liver function within the treated group, with no reports of adverse effects.

Likewise, when BMMSC were introduced intra-arterially in a canine liver fibrosis model, the procedure was deemed safe; however, it was observed that the decrease in liver enzyme levels lasted for a prolonged period when MSC were administered through intra-arterial means. [221]

Autologous ADMSCs were utilized intravenously multiple times to address degenerative hepatopathy in a group of ten dogs. Every animal displayed a remarkable enhancement in liver function, as evidenced by a decrease in hepatic biomarkers following each administration when compared to a control group. [222] A case study involving the treatment The discovery of hepatocutaneous syndrome being treated with mesenchymal stem cells was also recorded. Allogeneic adipose-derived mesenchymal stem cells were consistently delivered either through direct injection into liver tissue or intravenously. The outcome data showed a positive survival rate in dogs with improved or constrained clinical symptoms symptoms surpassed the anticipated outcome for this particular illness. [223].

IV administration of MSCs leads to the cells accumulating in the liver once they have been cleared from the lungs.[142] The intravenous route is considered a rational option for addressing liver diseases in animals that exhibit positive responses to mesenchymal stem cell therapy. Nonetheless, definitive statements regarding the most efficient method of administration, along with the efficacy and safety of using allogeneic mesenchymal stem cells for the treatment of liver diseases are constrained by the scarcity of research conducted on human subjects. Consequently, further investigation is essential to address these issues.

Conditions affecting the kidneys

Chronic kidney disease (CKD) is common in aging felines and is characterized by ongoing tubulointerstitial nephritis, tubular atrophy, and interstitial fibrosis. Currently, renal transplantation is the only available treatment that has the potential to restore kidney function. Chronic kidney disease (CKD) is common in aging felines and is characterized by ongoing tubulointerstitial nephritis, tubular atrophy, and interstitial fibrosis. Currently, renal transplantation is the only available treatment that has the potential to restore kidney function. [224].

Stem cell therapies present promising opportunities for less invasive treatment modalities. The transplantation of stem cells directly into the kidney poses dangers of significant adverse reactions and the need for anesthesia, thus highlighting intravenous infusion of stem cells as the preferred approach. Although the intravenous introduction of allogeneic adipose-derived mesenchymal stem cells in cats suffering from renal disease did not lead to any negative outcomes, there were no immediate enhancements noted in kidney function. [225-228].

Nevertheless, a study carried out by Vidane et al. [226] The study entailed the intravenous infusion of allogeneic mesenchymal stem cells derived from feline amniotic tissues into cats suffering from spontaneous chronic kidney disease. After the second dose of stem cells, a marked improvement in kidney function was observed. This progress was demonstrated by a lowering of serum creatinine and urine protein levels, as well as an elevation in urine concentration. Additionally, there was a notable enhancement in the cats' general clinical condition, including advancements in appetite and social interactions.

Cardiovascular disorders

In the field of human medicine, there has been a longstanding use of cardiac stem cell therapies aimed at repairing the myocardium in the aftermath of acute or chronic myocardial infarctions. The relentless advancement of this condition ultimately culminates in treatment-resistant congestive heart failure and mortality. [229-231].

In Dobermans, an experimental therapy was conducted utilizing retrograde coronary venous allogeneic ADMSC delivery to address this condition. It was determined that while the treatment was deemed safe, there were no significant positive outcomes resulting from the stem cell therapy. [232].

Within the domain of diminutive breeds of canines, the primary cardiac condition often observed is degenerative valvular disease, which commonly leads to issues such as ventricular enlargement and dysfunction. An investigation carried out by Petchdee and Sompeewong examined the effects of injecting stem cells intravenously derived from puppy deciduous teeth on this degenerative valvular disease.

The findings indicated enhancement in the left ventricular ejection fraction; however, it is important to note that this study was limited in scope, necessitating further research to substantiate any potential beneficial impacts. .[233, 234]

Conditions affecting the respiratory system

Respiratory issues are frequently encountered in veterinary medicine, particularly in horses, where diseases like asthma pose significant challenges due to the lack of highly effective treatment options. This disorder commonly originates from exposure to moldy hay, dusty straw, and various types of pollen. Symptoms in affected horses often include ongoing coughing, heightened difficulty breathing while at rest, and struggles with maintaining stamina during physical activity.

The clinical signs can be addressed through the administration of corticosteroids, bronchodilators, or modifications to the animal's environment.

It is important to note that medications may have undesirable side effects, necessitating the exploration of new therapeutic approaches. Barussi et al. conducted a study [235]

The results of their study indicated that the use of these cells led to enhancements, surpassing the benefits of dexamethasone treatment.

Additionally, there was an increase in IL-10 levels following the administration of cell therapy, which were significantly elevated in contrast to the control group that was given dexamethasone. These results align with positive outcomes observed in prior studies involving respiratory diseases in dogs and cats. [237].

Conditions affecting the neuromuscular system and resulting from injuries

Spinal cord injuries (SCI) are a prevalent neuromuscular condition affecting both humans and animals, often leading to permanent disabilities. In dogs, SCI can be caused by trauma or a herniated vertebral disc. Research has shown promising results in the treatment of these conditions with stem cell therapy. One study examined the use of autologous the administration of BMMSC therapy involved the local delivery of cells through hemilaminectomy. [238, 239].

In a separate research study, allogeneic Bone Marrow Mesenchymal Stem Cells (BMMSCs) were paired with standard medication therapy, resulting in a notably enhanced functional recovery among patients with traumatic spinal cord injury compared to those receiving only traditional medication. Another notable finding was the positive outcomes of MSC therapy in dogs with traumatic spinal cord injury and acute disc herniation. Dogs afflicted with acute paraplegia exhibited expedited improvement in mobility when administered epidural application of ADMSCs, in contrast to those undergoing solely surgical decompression.

Despite this, the introduction of autologous BMMSCs in dogs with degenerative intervertebral disc disease did not yield any enhancements in clinical results, nor did it demonstrate any regenerative impacts on the three dog patients examined. [240- 242].

Studies utilizing mesenchymal stem cells there were some favorable results observed in the treatment of traumatic spinal cord injuries and disc herniation in dogs ; however, further research is needed to enhance the therapeutic efficacy of MSC therapies currently observed.[243]

One potential avenue for improvement is through the utilization of a tissue engineering strategy. For example, in a particular study, a neural network tissue derived from canine MSCs was engineered and Implantation of cells into the spinal cord leads to the slowly returning motor function in paralyzed limbs. Further research must be carried out and progress made in this specialized area to ascertain the efficacy of cell therapy as well as tissue engineering methods for spinal cord injuries, particularly in cases of spontaneous injuries in patients that often exhibit a distinct disease progression from experimentally induced pathologies.

Conditions affecting the skin and the process of wound recovery

Unsuccessful wound healing can be attributed to a range of deficient cellular and molecular mechanisms, resulting in persistent, chronic wounds that cause discomfort for patients. Therefore, mesenchymal stem cells (MSCs) could serve as a promising treatment option for chronic wounds with severe inflammation and hyperplastic response, given their anti-inflammatory and regenerative properties. Numerous animal studies have demonstrated the advantageous in various species such as goats, sheep, horses, and dogs. [244-248].

In all four instances, successful results were noted through the development of scabs and minor marks at the core of the injury, ultimately promoting tissue proliferation within a month following treatment. Additionally, a separate scenario entailed the total recovery of a persistent skin wound in a juvenile horse after multiple administrations of Heterologous mesenchymal stem cells derived from Wharton's Jelly, when paired with a carboxymethylcellulose gel, resulted in the rapid attainment of complete wound closure within a span of just five days. [249].

The initial study did not show any notable improvement in clinical symptoms or itchiness. However, the second study, which involved 22 dogs with atopic dermatitis unresponsive to traditional therapies, demonstrated a significant reduction in itchiness after one week and improvement in cadesi-04 scores after one month following intravenous administration of allogeneic MSCs. The remission of clinical symptoms persisted for a minimum of six months, with no adverse reactions reported. [259-251].

Multiple research studies conducted on both laboratory animals and clinical veterinary patients indicate that stem cells could potentially serve as an innovative therapy to facilitate the healing of chronic wounds. However, similar to other medical conditions, there are still numerous unanswered questions that must be investigated in forthcoming studies before these treatments can be integrated into standard clinical practice. The current data pertaining to using stem cells to treat AD in dogs is extremely limited, making it challenging to determine if such treatments may provide benefits in the future.

Eye Diseases

Research is being conducted on the use of stem cell therapy in the field of ophthalmology. Certain eye conditions, such as corneal ulcers, currently lack effective treatments. In a series of clinical cases involving horses, Autologous peripheral blood stem cells were employed to treat chronic corneal ulcers and retinal detachment that had proven resistant to conventional therapies.

These cells were delivered either via intravenous infusion or locally through techniques such as subconjunctival injection or eye drop application. Subsequent to the treatment, all four individuals demonstrated marked progress, notably in the closure of the epithelial surface and alleviation of inflammation. [37].

In 75% of horses, the administration of autologous bone marrow-derived mesenchymal stem cells directly into the subconjunctiva led to an improvement in immune-mediated keratitis, resulting in enhanced corneal clarity, reduced neovascularization, and minimized surface irregularities.

Additionally, the immune-modulating properties of MSCs have the potential to alter the progression of equine recurrent uveitis as demonstrated by a decrease in interferon-gamma expression by cd4+ T cells from ERU-affected horses upon exposure to adipose-derived mesenchymal stem cells in vitro. The activation of CD4+ T cells was also observed to decrease through a contact-dependent mechanism and signaling mediated by prostaglandin E2 [252, 253].

Mesenchymal stem cell therapy is being considered for the treatment of feline eosinophilic keratitis in cats. Research indicates that allogeneic adipose-derived MSCs, when implanted subconjunctivally, exhibited encouraging outcomes in reducing the clinical manifestations of FEK progressively [254]

In dogs, MSC therapy has emerged as a viable therapeutic option for keratoconjunctivitis sicca (KCS) or dry eye disease. Another study revealed that implanting allogeneic adipose-derived MSCs locally around the lacrimal gland of both eyes led to a significant reduction in clinical signs, with this effect being sustained throughout the study period.

Furthermore, research by Sgrignoli et al. [255] after six months of consistently applying allogeneic ADMSCs to the conjunctival sac, a noticeable decrease was observed in the levels of KCS markers including CD4, IL-6, IL-1, and TNF-α in canines. [256]

Based on research findings, Mesenchymal Stem Cell (MSC) therapy has emerged as a promising approach in the realm of regenerative ophthalmology, presenting novel remedies for a range of eye ailments in animals including corneal ulcers, immune-mediated and eosinophilic keratitis, recurrent uveitis, and dry keratoconjunctivitis. Nonetheless, additional double-blind prospective trials, specifically focusing on recurrent uveitis in equines, are imperative for a more precise assessment of the real-world effectiveness of MSC therapy.

It is evident that ongoing scientific investigation is essential in order to gain a comprehensive understanding of the intricacies and seriousness of specific eye diseases, as well as the regenerative properties of stem cells in ocular therapies. This knowledge could ultimately facilitate the advancement of stem cell therapy towards clinical application.

Diseases affecting the reproductive system

Numerous research studies are being conducted in an effort to discover potential treatments aimed at enhancing fertility, particularly with applications in the agricultural sector for livestock and potential translation into human medical practices. Despite efforts aimed at restoring fertility through the intraovarian injection of BMMSC, the desired outcome of improved ovarian function in aging mares could not be achieved. [257]. Similarly, there were no observed alterations in sperm characteristics or fertility rates following intratesticular administration of allogeneic Bone Marrow Mesenchymal Stem Cells (BMMSC) in horses. Nonetheless, the proven safety of this method implies the potential for utilizing it in the treatment of degenerative conditions affecting the testes. [258].

Interestingly, the treatment of dog sperm with ADMSC derived ECV during cryopreservation appears to be effective, as the addition of ECVs resulted in a reduction of damaged sperm and decreased levels of ROS in thawed semen. There is a promising potential for MSC treatment to address pathologies of reproductive organs, based on the outcomes of treating other inflammatory conditions. For instance, endometriosis in mares is a degenerative disease of the uterus that poses significant economic challenges in the equine industry.

In order to capitalize on the immunomodulatory abilities of MSCs in uterine disorders, researchers have examined and separated endometrial MSCs from a range of animal species such as sows, cows, ewes, goats, and mares. Mambelli et al. have suggested administering MSCs to the uterus of mares with endometriosis, showing that these cells can remain present in the uterus for as long as 21 days following intrauterine administration. [259- 266]

Further examination is needed to evaluate the potential immunomodulatory and anti-inflammatory characteristics of endometrial MSCs and their efficacy in treating endometriosis. Not only are investigations underway for the use of MSC therapy in addressing reproductive system disorders, but current research is also exploring its application in treating mastitis in livestock.

Studies have demonstrated a suppressive impact on Staphylococcus aureus-induced mastitis in cows and have indicated that it can facilitate healing and reduce fibrosis in cases of chronic mastitis in goats. [267, 268].

The safety and regulatory implications associated with the utilization of stem cell therapies in veterinary medicine.

Vigilant monitoring of the entire production process, starting from material sourcing up to the final product, is crucial from a microbiological perspective. With the rising utilization of allogeneic mesenchymal stem cell (MSC) therapies in dogs and horses, new concerns arise for manufacturers, regulatory bodies, and end-users.

As of now, there is a lack of specific directives in this area.

Furthermore, the necessity of investigating protozoa in dogs and horses may vary based on the geographical origin of the animals, prevalent epidemiological factors in that region.

Moreover, it is strongly advised that individuals who provide cell donations uphold a state of good health as a standardized practice. When working with cells sourced from newly born animals or placental tissues, it is prudent to conduct screenings on mothers with the aim of detecting any potential infectious pathogens. It is critical to confirm the absence of pathogenic agents by means of a thorough procedure that includes donor evaluations based on medical background and clinical information, testing donors for specific pathogens, and scrutinizing the final cell product for potential impurities.

Additionally, maintaining a sterile manufacturing environment is essential for reducing the risk of introducing foreign agents. [269].

Currently, there is no uniform legislation within the European Union pertaining to the use of stem cell therapies in veterinary medicine. As a result, each member state of the EU governs this field independently. However, it is anticipated that this situation will soon change, as the European Medicines Agency

(EMA) is set to issue guidelines and regulatory frameworks for regenerative veterinary medicine.

Such products must undergo a premarket review process in order to be approved for legal distribution.

To obtain approval for market distribution, these cell-based products must demonstrate safety, efficacy, and manufacturing quality [48].

In the coming years, we anticipate the implementation of additional regulatory guidelines. The impact of these new regulations on the progress of stem cell trials and the creation of innovative therapies remains uncertain. It is imperative that any forthcoming regulations are crafted and endorsed by a panel of experts spanning diverse fields, from cell biology to clinical veterinary medicine.

Presently, there are no animal cell-based treatments that have received approval from the FDA. Recognizing the immense potential of veterinary regenerative medicine [270].

The central importance of stem cells in the realms of veterinary regenerative medicine and tissue engineering.

The main objective of tissue engineering is the regeneration of impaired tissues and their substitution with fully functional ones, thereby enabling the restoration of their complete functionality. This intricate process involves a multidisciplinary approach, requiring expertise in various fields such as the disciplines constitute areas of study within the field of biological sciences. [271].

For many years, researchers have explored various therapeutic options in various animal models and research levels to be utilized in regenerative therapy for both animals and humans. [272,277]. Despite this, stem cells remain a topic of great interest in the scientific community, being identified as cells capable of self-renewal and differentiation. [278,279].

From the moment of fertilization of the ovum until the point of demise, these cells can be found within all organisms. Their presence is crucial for the growth of tissues and the maintenance of the balance of somatic cells. Furthermore, they facilitate the regeneration of organs and tissues by replacing somatic cells that age or experience damage. [280] The longstanding goal of humanity to replace damaged or deteriorating cells and tissues with newly generated ones in a controlled laboratory environment. These iPSCs are altered somatic cells that acquire the characteristics of stem cells. [281].

It is currently feasible to utilize stem cells in both human and veterinary medicine due to extensive research conducted across various scientific disciplines. Various researchers have highlighted the unique attributes of stem cells, including their uncomplicated structure and limited specialization, ability to self-renew and maintain a continuous cell population throughout an organism's lifespan, asymmetric division resulting in two stem cells of different sizes with one undergoing further differentiation, capability to differentiate into various tissue types, and expression of specific proteins. [278,284-286].

This publication contains a comprehensive overview of the current knowledge on the utilization of stem cells in veterinary medicine. The content is derived from selected scientific studies and addresses various types of stem cells, their immunomodulatory attributes, and an evaluation of the effectiveness of this therapy in treating a range of medical conditions in animals, including those affecting the heart, skin, digestive system, musculoskeletal system, kidneys, respiratory system, and eyes.

Stem Cells Classification

Stem cells are characterized as cells that remain undifferentiated and can be found in various life stages, from embryonic to adult, where they give rise to the mature cells that form different tissues and organs in the body. These cells are categorized according to different factors such as their ability to differentiate, their source, and their compatibility with the host. [287].

Differentiation Potential

When examining the potential differentiation capabilities of stem cells, they have the capacity to exhibit a range of characteristics such as totipotent, pluripotent, multipotent, oligo-/bipotent, or unipotent. Totipotent stem cells showcase an unlimited ability for proliferation.

These cells possess a unique potential to transform into any cell type involved in the formation of embryonic and extra-embryonic tissues (such as the placenta and umbilical cord), thereby enabling the formation of a complete organism. Studies on monozygotic twins originating from multiple blastomeres indicate that the fertilized ovum (zygote) serves as the totipotent cell, with cells stemming from the initial germinal stage (morula). [288,289].

In contrast to totipotent cells, they do not have the capability to give rise to all the tissues present in the body. An example of pluripotent cells can be found in the blastocyst germ cells, alternatively referred to as the inner cell mass (ICM). Multipotent cells exhibit a remarkable capacity to differentiate into diverse cell types originating from a singular germ layer emerges cells known as germ layer-derived cells. This is depicted in Figure 1.

Mesenchymal stem cells possess a distinctive ability to proliferate extensively, differentiate into a variety of cell types from different sources, and interact with the host organism.

Among the various types of stem cells, mesenchymal stem cells have received the most attention from researchers. Oligo-/bipotent stem cells are characterized by their ability to differentiate into multiple lineages within a specific tissue. [287,293].

The swine ocular cells have showcased proficiency in generating conjunctival and corneal cells. Unipotent stem cells, also referred to as precursor cells, display a distinctive differentiation process that leads to the formation of a specific mature cell type. Such differentiation is evident in the germinal layer cells of the epidermis, as they play a role in preserving a constant cell count in tissues under usual conditions. [294].

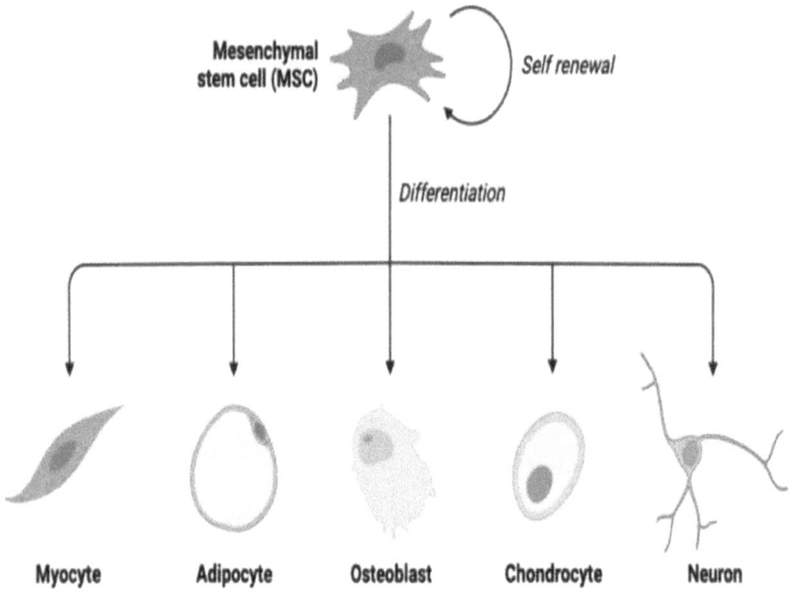

Figure 1

Illustration depicting the capability of mesenchymal stem cells to differentiate into multiple cell types

Origin of Stem Cells

Based on their source, stem cells can be categorized as embryonic, adult, tissue-derived, or iPSCs. Totipotent embryonic stem cells (ESCs) are derived from the blastomeres of the embryo. However, the pluripotent cells most frequently used in research come from the blastocyst embryonic node. Fetal stem cells (FSCs) can be obtained from fetal tissues, umbilical cord tissues like Wharton's jelly, umbilical cord blood, and amniotic cells. [295].

Embryonic stem cells possess an infinite ability to regenerate and transform into various cell types in a controlled environment. However, currently there has not been a successful method developed to regulate their differentiation and proliferation at the point of injection within a living organism, potentially leading to the development of cancerous growths observed in experimental subjects. These obstacles, in addition to ethical considerations, have significantly impeded the application of ESCs in medical stem cell therapies. Somatic or mature cells, also known as adult stem cells, are distinguished by their restricted ability to differentiate into multiple or single cell types. [296, 297]

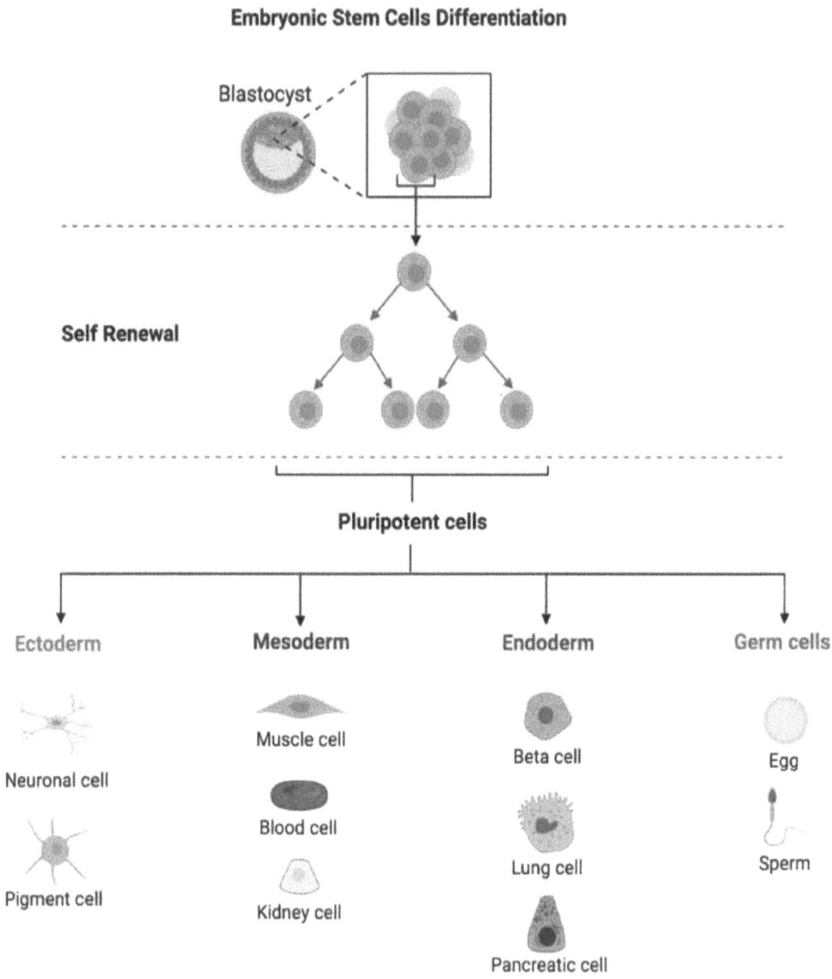

Figure 2

Illustration of the origin and various pathways of differentiation for embryonic stem cells.

The maintenance of tissues and organs in the body following birth is contingent upon their presence during the postnatal period. Instead of depending on pluripotent cells obtained from embryos, autologous stem cells with pluripotent capabilities can be generated by reprogramming adult somatic cells, like fibroblasts, within a well-regulated laboratory setting.

Through the introduction of key genes essential for embryonic cell development, these reprogrammed cells are generated. It is worth noting that the resulting induced pluripotent stem cells have the capacity to differentiate in a manner akin to embryonic cells. However, this method has shown limited success, as laboratory mice injected with these cells developed teratomas. [298].

Connection to the receiver

Stem cells are categorized into autologous, allogeneic, or xenogeneic types based on their relationship to the recipient, as stated by researchers [299]. Autogenic cells, currently the focus of much research, are derived from the recipient animal, which also serves as the donor. [299].

Allogeneic stem cells offer a convenient option for regenerative therapy, allowing for immediate use and avoiding the time-consuming process of culturing autologous cells. Nevertheless, the primary limitation of allogeneic stem cells is the necessity for a donor. Xenogeneic stem cells serve as a potential alternative to both autologous and allogeneic stem cells. [300].

Xenogeneic stem cells can be obtained and isolated from a range of animals from diverse species. Numerous research findings utilizing antlerogenic (xenogeneic) cells have indicated that specific species, including rabbits and horses, possess the capability for stem cell retrieval [301], The subjects demonstrated a rejuvenating reaction [302].

Potential origins of mesenchymal stem cells within bodily tissues

Research has revealed that the type of cells, determined by their source, greatly impacts their capacity for in vivo differentiation and their key physiological traits. [296]. When deciding on the origin of MSCs for a specific therapy, it is important to carefully consider which source to utilize. Bone marrow is a widely studied source of MSCs in veterinary care, mirroring its use in human medicine. [303- 305].

Regrettably, the collection of samples in animals involves invasive procedures carried out during the administration of general anesthetics in dogs and sedatives, with or without local anesthetics, in horses, can lead to postoperative complications such as infection and/or bleeding. Various studies have documented cases of inadvertent cardio-thoracic punctures and instances of pneumopericardium in horses.[306, 307]

However, the procedure for collecting BM-MSC from these animals can be safely performed on a standing animal, minimizing the risks associated with previous methods. It is now widely accepted that the most suitable location for sternal biopsy using a Jamshidi needle is at the 4th or 5th sternebra. As animals age, the quantity of BM-MSCs decreases, representing a small fraction of all bone marrow stromal mononuclear cells. The aspirate extracted the donor's contribution is employed for cultivating and advancing MSCs in a laboratory setting. The effectiveness of MSCs in therapy is closely linked to the quantity of cultured MSCs, with a maximum capacity of four passages. The culture process involves several stages, including establishment of the culture, cell proliferation, medium changing, and final determination.[308-311]

In recent times, there has been growing interest in utilizing adipose tissue as a viable source for extracting and isolating mesenchymal stem cells (MSCs). A common method for acquiring this material involves performing during preventative ovariohysterectomy procedures in dogs and cats, a scheduled removal of fat tissue, known as lipectomy or lipoaspiration, is conducted. This fat tissue includes both subcutaneous and visceral fat, which are recognized as potential reservoirs of adipose-derived mesenchymal stem cells (AD-MSCs).

Following collection, a small number of nucleated cells exhibiting AD-MSC characteristics can be extracted from the aspirate. Similar to bone marrow-derived MSCs (BM-MSCs), it is imperative to culture these fat-derived cells in a controlled laboratory setting in order to achieve a therapeutic dosage. [312, 313]

Specialized laboratory procedures, including enzymatic breakdown, sequential rinsing, and centrifugation, are necessary for this process. AD-MSCs have shown a remarkable capacity for both differentiation and proliferation, making them a commonly utilized cell source in regenerative medicine. These cells are frequently utilized in the treatment of musculoskeletal disorders, boasting greater accessibility and ease of acquisition compared to BM-MSCs. [314,315].

PB-MSCs, considered as an alternative source of MSCs, are the subject of discussion. The method of collecting a blood sample, which is considered the safest and least controversial, is preferred due to its effectiveness compared to other methods.

An investigation conducted by scientists revealed that only 30% of the test horses exhibited a satisfactory level of blood cells for subsequent cell cultivation. Moreover, specialized interventions, including hyperbaric chambers, were employed to enhance the number of PB-MSCs in the peripheral circulation of these creatures. [316-318].

It is widely acknowledged that the efficacy of mesenchymal stem cells diminishes with the age of the donor. Cells derived from fetal tissues have demonstrated the ability to differentiate not only into mesenchymal cells but also cells from the other three germ layers, indicating their pluripotent nature. The minimally invasive process of obtaining these tissues occurs during the perinatal period, in contrast to the collection of bone marrow-derived mesenchymal stem cells or adipose tissue-derived mesenchymal stem cells. However, the method of material acquisition may have limitations in terms of sterility. [319-322].

MSCs from the same individual, from a different individual, and from a different species

The ongoing discussion among experts at a global level focuses on the discrepancy in safety and effectiveness in the use of these cells for therapeutic purposes. As previously mentioned, Mesenchymal Stem Cells (MSCs) can be classified based on their origin as allogeneic, autologous, or xenogeneic, depending on the relationship between the donor and the recipient. Allogeneic cells are those that are transferred from one donor to a recipient of the same species. In comparison to autologous cells, the efficient cultivation of allogeneic cells in a controlled setting significantly reduces the time required for treatment. MIC-1 stem cells, derived from deer and falling under the allogeneic category, were therapeutically utilized in horses and experimentally injected into the tissues of injured rabbits. [323].

Due to interspecies differences between donors and recipients, the use of mesenchymal stem cells (MSCs) from animals is not common. Researchers are actively evaluating the effectiveness of allogeneic versus autologous cells in regenerative medicine and exploring alternative treatment options. Careful consideration of the pros and cons of each MSC type is crucial when selecting the appropriate therapy. Ideally, MSCs obtained directly from the same organism would be the most secure source. Consequently, autologous cells are generally considered a safer choice for therapy; however, the process of harvesting Generating an ample supply of these cells can be a labor-intensive process that may necessitate surgical intervention, entailing potential complications such as infection and disease transmission. [324].

The method is occasionally used due to the above-mentioned challenges and the high cost associated with the procedure. Various variables such as the age, gender, and type of illness of an animal play a crucial role in determining the abundance and caliber of self-derived cells in the organism. Conversely, cells from unrelated donors can be grown and preserved in a cellular repository for an indefinite period. This practice allows for the consistent identification of the quantity of MSCs, safety standards, and potential for differentiation in a single-cell batch. [325-327].

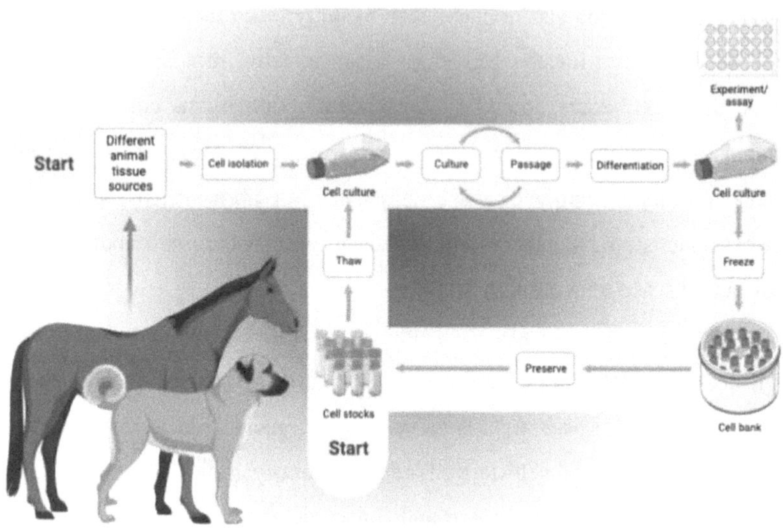

Figure 3
Representation of the workflow of autologous and allogeneic mesenchymal stem cells, including processes such as harvesting, culturing, storage, and utilization, presented in a schematic manner.

Employing such a strategy would result in a reduction of the time needed for collecting materials and cultivating cells, while also minimizing typical variability as seen in autogenic cells. It would further promote uniformity in therapeutic applications and expected outcomes. It is crucial to adhere to national legal standards governing the use of medical preparations, particularly when working with allogeneic cells. Bertoni and colleagues conducted a study investigating the effects of autologous research conducted on the fetlocks of healthy horses using allogeneic stem cells has produced interesting results. While there were no significant alterations in the synovial fluid properties, it was noted that the use of BM-MSCs led to a noticeable increase in synovial effusion compared to UCB-MSCs. Furthermore, MSC injections resulted in mild to moderate local inflammatory reactions, with a greater reduction in inflammation evident in more cells during clinical and ultrasonographic assessments. [327- 329].

Evidence of the acceptance of allogeneic stem cells is demonstrated through the existence of two allogeneic cell therapy products for equines and one for canines have obtained marketing authorization from the European Medicines Agency, alongside others. Numerous studies have examined the application of xenogeneic stem cells, utilizing various experimental animals including rodents, lagomorphs, canines, and primates for both local and systemic cultivation of these cells. Research on rats has shown that xenogeneic cells (murine) were still detectable in the bone marrow 12 weeks after being introduced into the carotid artery. Apart from the bone marrow, these cells have also been observed in myocardial infarction tissue as immature myocytes, indicating their potential for therapeutic use in various medical conditions. [330-332].

Several recent studies have demonstrated the efficacy of utilizing xenogeneic cells for various medical treatments. For example, experiments involving rat stem cells have successfully regenerated In rabbits, bone tissue has been found to exhibit significant potential for regenerative medicine applications, whereas promising outcomes have been observed in the use of human bone marrow stem cells for the treatment of spinal cord injuries in rats. [333-335].

MSCs have the ability to modulate the immune system

Recipient CD8+ T cells have the capability to detect foreign cells bearing MHC I surface proteins, thus eliciting a direct cytotoxic effect on these cells. Furthermore, recipient CD4+ T cells can target cells expressing MHC II molecules, triggering either a cytotoxic or humoral immune response. B cells, when identified indirectly by antigen-presenting cells, have the potential to generate alloantibodies. [336].

Although there is limited data available regarding their immunogenicity, it is widely believed that adult MSCs have low immunogenicity. This is primarily due to the absence of MHC II antigens on their surface and the limited expression of MHC I. Adult MSCs have the ability to inhibit the proliferation and normal function of NK cells, T lymphocytes, and B lymphocytes. They also have the capacity to suppress antigen-presenting cells support the generation of suppressor T cells. [337].

Mesenchymal stem cells (MSCs) only exhibit MHC I molecules on their surface upon differentiation into adipogenic, osteogenic, and chondrogenic lineages. This observation implies that allogeneic MSCs could potentially be utilized as a convenient reservoir for regenerative therapy in veterinary medicine, given their supposed immune privilege.

However, it is crucial to acknowledge the potential risk of disease transmission from the donor to the recipient. Therefore, a specialized systemic approach must be implemented to manage possible viral, bacterial, and fungal infections specific to each species.

Studies have indicated that the secretome is generally safer than MSCs themselves, even when administered in high doses, with minimal adverse effects. Moreover, it shows a lower propensity for emboli formation following intravenous administration and a reduced risk of Pathological or tumorigenic alterations are observed when comparing them to the changes linked to uncontrolled cell differentiation. [338-341].

Utilizing Stem Cells for Regeneration and Bioengineering Purposes in Various Body Organs and Tissues within Veterinary Medicine

Stem cells have been utilized mainly on an experimental level to treat a diverse array of diseases in various animal species. Initially, the veterinary field focused on using regenerative medicine for orthopedic conditions, but there is now a rapid expansion to include other ailments like those impacting Stem cells. Additionally, cats with kidney and respiratory issues, as well as various inflammatory conditions, have also benefited from treatment with these cells. [296].

Heart

Cardiovascular diseases have emerged as the primary cause of mortality in the global human population. Similarly, these diseases present a significant threat to animals, often with cases going unnoticed.

This technological advancement holds the potential to enhance the timely identification of issues and subsequently guide patients towards appropriate treatment modalities [342 - 351].

Several years ago, cardiac stem cell treatments Stem cell therapy has been employed in the field of human medicine to mend damaged myocardium caused by both sudden and chronic myocardial infarctions. While primary myocardial infarctions are uncommon in companion animals, dilated cardiomyopathy is frequently observed in larger dog breeds. This condition typically worsens over time, ultimately resulting in irreversible congestive heart failure and death. To explore potential treatments, an experimental approach involving the delivery of allogeneic AD-MSCs through the retrograde coronary venous route was conducted on Dobermans with dilated cardiomyopathy. [352].

Degenerative valve disease is a frequently observed cardiac ailment in smaller canine breeds often leading to ventricular enlargement and cardiac dysfunction. A study by Petchdee and Sompeewong explored for treating degenerative valvular conditions, showing some improvement in left ventricular ejection fraction in a small trial. Further research is essential to validate any positive outcomes observed in this preliminary study. [353].

Skin

Inadequate cellular and molecular pathways often interfere with the successful healing of wounds, leading to the development of persistent, chronic wounds that cause discomfort to the affected animal. Mesenchymal stem cells (MSCs) have shown promise as a potential therapy. Research has shown the beneficial impact of MSC therapy on wound healing in various animal models such as caprines, ovines, horses, and canines, highlighting its potential effectiveness in treating chronic wounds. [354- 357].

Extracellular vesicles (ECVs) produced by mesenchymal stem cells (MSCs) were employed to enhance the healing of dogs' wounds when injected locally, resulting in significantly improved cutaneous wound healing. Another study involved the topical and systemic administration of peripheral blood stem cells (PBSCs) to four horses with spontaneous infected wounds that were unresponsive to conventional therapies. All four cases demonstrated tissue expansion after four weeks of treatment, evidenced by the formation of scabs and small scars at the incision site. [382-383].

Further investigation revealed the successful healing of a chronic skin wound in a young female horse using repeated applications of stem cells derived from umbilical cord Wharton's jelly, with the assistance of carboxymethylcellulose gel. Within just 5 days, the wound had fully healed. In contrast, these stem cells were also utilized in the treatment of atopic dermatitis in dogs, a common skin condition, as well as for wound healing.

Research on laboratory and clinical veterinary animals suggests that stem cells could be a promising avenue for supporting chronic wound healing. However, numerous challenges need to be addressed through further research before these therapies can be widely implemented in clinical settings.

Due to a lack of comprehensive information on atopic dermatitis in dogs, it is currently difficult to predict the effectiveness of stem cell therapies for this condition [384- 386]

Digestive System

Mouth and Teeth

The animal's overall well-being can be greatly affected by oral discomfort and issues with chewing. In recent times, oral and dental problems have become increasingly common in dogs and cats across the globe, leading to significant pain and the risk of infections. Stem cells have emerged as a promising option for repairing oral and dental tissues through regenerative cell therapy. Research has highlighted the potential of mesenchymal stem cells (MSCs) in regulating The immune responses are instrumental in promoting the recovery of both periodontal and dental tissues, while also aiding in the augmentation of healing processes for implants [387-389].

In the miniature pig model used to study periodontal defects, the use of allogeneic AD-MSCs has shown potential in stimulating the regeneration of periodontal tissue. Studies have emphasized the effectiveness of both autologous and allogeneic dental pulp stem cells, as well as autogenous BM-MSCs, in the restoration of canine dental pulp. These findings indicate the possibility of regenerating oro-dental tissues, despite varying perspectives on the efficacy of stem cells in treating dental conditions, such as issues with dental implants. [390, 391].

Research using animal models is essential for establishing a foundational framework and standard for the progress of stem cell and tissue engineering methods aimed at enhancing the regeneration of orodental tissues.

Further investigation is required to fully assess the effectiveness and significance of stem cell treatments for addressing oro-dental problems in animals with inherent disorders. Feline chronic gingivostomatitis (FCGS) is a painful oral condition commonly seen in cats, distinguished by chronic inflammation of the gums that spreads to the buccal and caudal oral mucosa. The primary symptoms of FCGS include loss of appetite, oral pain, weight loss, increased drooling, bad breath, and reduced grooming habits. [392].

Presently, treatment options for Feline Chronic Gingivostomatitis (FCGS) encompass the use of corticosteroids, cyclosporin, and tooth extraction surgery. These treatments have shown different response rates and are associated with various potential side effects. The utilization of Mesenchymal Stem Cell (MSC) therapy in FCGS has demonstrated notably favorable outcomes. IV therapy using autologous Adipose-Derived MSCs has resulted in complete presentation in most felines [393-397].

Allogeneic adipose-derived mesenchymal stem cells have been noted to demonstrate reduced clinical effectiveness in comparison to autologous MSCs for the management of feline chronic gingivostomatitis. A majority of cats afflicted with FCGS who received intravenous allogeneic adipose-derived MSCs exhibited signs of improvement in terms of clinical, histopathological, and systemic response, with around 70% displaying positive outcomes. [299].

Gastrointestinal Tract refers to the system of organs responsible for processing food and extracting nutrients

Recurrent gastrointestinal symptoms accompanied by evidence of inflammation and of unknown etiology. [399,400]. Some dogs show resistance to conventional treatments like cyclosporine or steroids. A study found that nine out of 11 dogs suffering from severe inflammatory bowel disease achieved clinical remission after receiving a single intravenous infusion of allogenic adipose-derived mesenchymal stem cells six weeks post-treatment. Additionally, there was a significant improvement. [361].

In cats, Inflammatory Bowel Disease is a common condition characterized by frequent bouts of vomiting and diarrhea. A study involving the use of Allogeneic Adipose-Derived Mesenchymal Stem Cells in cats with IBD showed promising results. Conversely, cats who received a placebo showed no improvement and may have experienced a worsening of their condition.

Due to their immunomodulatory and anti-inflammatory properties, MSCs are being considered as a potential alternative therapy for IBD in both dogs and cats. While the initial findings of the study are positive, further research and larger studies are necessary to determine the safety and efficacy of MSC therapy for treating IBD in animals [362].

Liver

Additionally, a separate research study employed mesenchymal stem cells in an experimental model focusing on liver cirrhosis in canines.

The findings revealed that the intravenous infusion of autologous bone marrow-derived MSCs notably decreased hepatic fibrosis, leading to positive enhancements in liver function among the treated subjects. [363- 364].

In a study using dogs to simulate liver fibrosis, it was found that intra-arterial administration of bone marrow-derived mesenchymal stem cells (BM-MSCs) proved to be safe, comparable to intravenous administration. Surprisingly, those dogs that received intra-arterial injections of MSCs exhibited a longer-lasting reduction in liver enzyme levels in the blood.

Furthermore, a separate experiment involved treating ten dogs with degenerative hepatopathy with intravenous injections of autologous adipose tissue-derived mesenchymal stem cells (AD-MSCs) on a recurring basis. When compared to a control group, all the treated animals displayed significant improvements in liver function, indicated by reductions in hepatic biomarkers after each round of treatment [401, 402].

Moreover, a case study involving the treatment of hepato-cutaneous syndrome with mesenchymal stem cells (MSCs) was presented. In this study, allogeneic adipose-derived MSCs were administered intravenously or directly into the liver tissue. The outcomes indicated that in cases of this syndrome, dogs treated with MSCs exhibited prolonged survival despite experiencing relapsed or limited clinical symptoms, surpassing expectations. The intravenous route of administration appears to be a viable option for addressing hepatic conditions responsive to MSC therapy in animals. This is supported by the observation that

MSCs injected intravenously are able to accumulate in the liver following clearance from the lungs. The limited number of trials conducted on clinical cases poses challenges in determining the most optimal delivery method, as well as assessing the safety and efficacy of allogeneic MSCs for treating hepatic disorders. Consequently, further research is necessary to address these issues. [403, 404]

Musculoskeletal System

Tendons and Ligaments

Injuries to tendons and ligaments, whether caused by trauma or stress, typically heal through the formation Scar tissue, which is inferior to healthy tissue, forms as a result of the initial injury. This leads to a reduction in the structural integrity and disrupts the natural architecture and function of the tendon or ligament. Consequently, the locomotor function is impaired and more susceptible to additional injuries. Therefore, the main goal of treatment should be to regain the original structure and function of the tissue.

Conventional therapies for addressing tendon injuries in equines typically involve the application of cold therapy, wrapping the injured area with bandages, and implementing a period of rest before gradually increasing physical activity. In certain circumstances, corticosteroids or other anti-inflammatory medications may be prescribed as part of the treatment plan; nevertheless, surgical intervention is frequently necessary to effectively resolve the ailment. [405- 408].

With these conservative methods, reinjury is common and animals often struggle to regain their pre-injury level of function. The optimal approach to treatment, therefore, should prioritize the regeneration of the tendon matrix. In light of its potential for enhancing tissue regeneration, the utilization of mesenchymal stem cells has been suggested as an alternative to traditional methods.

Thus, stem cells derived from tendons would be the preferred source for regenerating tendon injuries, although extracting stem cells from tendon tissue poses significant challenges and there currently exists no established protocol for stimulating tendon regeneration. [410].

Hence, in the pursuit of restoring tendons, various sources of stem cells have been utilized, with an emphasis on adipose tissue and bone marrow. In the year 2003, the pioneering practice of autologous bone marrow-derived mesenchymal stem cell (BM-MSC) transplantation was introduced in the treatment of superficial digital flexor tendon injuries in horses. Promising outcomes were observed in a study involving the injection of cells into 11 racehorses with such injuries. Additionally, a study on 141 racehorses with naturally occurring superficial digital flexor tendon injuries revealed a reinjury rate of at least 28% following intralesional administration of autologous BM-MSCs. [411-414].

Nevertheless, in comparison to alternative treatments like platelet-rich plasma (PRP), autologous bone marrow- or adipose-derived mesenchymal stem cell therapy demonstrated minimal to negligible improvement in surgically induced lesions of the superficial digital flexor tendons in horses. [415-423].

Joints

The regenerative potential of cartilage tissue is constrained by its sparse cell population and absence of vascular supply. In equines, this constraint is worsened by the significant mechanical strain and pressure endured by the joint surfaces during physical activity. Problems with joints, specifically osteoarthritis, frequently lead to the premature termination of horses' competitive careers and enduring lameness. The success of conventional therapies for musculoskeletal disorders that impact cartilage, ligaments, and menisci is often influenced by the athletic capabilities of horses. [424-426].

Studies conducted in living organisms have demonstrated the effectiveness of intra-articular mesenchymal stem cell therapy in treating horses with ailments related to cartilage, bone, and the meniscus. One example of such a condition is bone spavin, which is a progressive degenerative disorder affecting the joints. commonly treated with corticosteroids, is a well-researched ailment in the equine locomotor system.

A study involving 16 horses with bone spavin demonstrated the positive and long-lasting effects of intraarticular AD-MSC treatment.

After a period of 180 days following the treatment, it was observed that the horses treated with MSCs did not experience lameness, unlike the control group. Scintigraphy results indicated the absence of inflammation in the treated tarsal joints, in contrast to the joints still showing signs of inflammation in the control group. in the control group. In cases of meniscal injury in horses, MSC therapy has shown promise, with a higher success rate in returning horses to work compared to arthroscopy alone. [427].

In a particular study, allogeneic AD-MSCs were utilized in the treatment of 80 horses suffering from osteoarthritis. Over the 90-day monitoring period, a significant reduction in lameness was observed, showcasing the beneficial effects of allogeneic cells. Likewise, comparable outcomes were demonstrated in horses treated with allogeneic UC-MSCs for metacarpophalangeal/metatarsophalangeal osteoarthritis. However, there was a lack of substantial clinical improvement after a 6-month period. It has been noted in various investigations that repetitive administration of allogeneic MSCs to osteoarthritic horses led to adverse clinical responses [428]. After receiving just one injection, allogeneic Mesenchymal Stem Cells have been documented to induce mild to moderate local inflammatory reactions [329].

Based on various research studies involving dogs, the introduction of MSCs into arthritic joints has been shown to alleviate pain and enhance functionality in animals.

The substantial decrease in lameness observed in dogs with stifle osteoarthritis following treatment with autologous AD-MSCs, as opposed to a placebo, suggests a markedly slower progression of the disease in the joints treated with the former [429]. Black and colleagues [430] along with Vilar and colleagues [319] found similar results in dogs suffering from hip osteoarthritis. Through research spanning up to four years, it has been shown that the benefits of using autologous adipose-derived mesenchymal stem cells (AD-MSCs) via intra-articular administration for treating osteoarthritis in various joints in dogs seem to have enduring effects. [431].

The use of allogeneic AD-MSCs has proven to vastly improve MSC therapy for osteoarthritis. Research on 74 dogs treated with allogeneic AD-MSCs showed no adverse effects, unlike the placebo group, and demonstrated a reduction in clinical symptoms. [432-433].

In an experimental model of osteoarthritis in dogs treated with allogeneic umbilical cord-derived mesenchymal stem cells, there was notable evidence of cartilage repair when compared to the control group.

This repair process included cartilage regeneration, decreased joint fluid, reduced inflammation, and improved healing of neighboring tissues. Unlike studies in horses, it has been shown that multiple injections of allogeneic mesenchymal stem cell therapy is safe for canine patients, with minimal and temporary inflammatory reactions and no adverse effects reported even after two years post-treatment. [434-435].

Research has been conducted on the efficacy of both autologous and allogeneic mesenchymal stem cell (MSC) therapies in treating canine osteoarthritis, with promising results observed when these treatments are combined with platelet-rich plasma (PRP) or hyaluronic acid.

Research has indicated that MSC therapy in combination with PRP yielded more robust and favorable results in the treatment of osteoarthritis in dogs. Extracellular vesicle (ECV) treatment has been successfully utilized in the management of suspensory ligament injuries in equines, showcasing impressive outcomes [436-437].

Muscles and Nerves

Spinal cord injuries, a significant cause of permanent disability, are common neuromuscular injuries in both humans and animals. In dogs, such injuries can occur as a result of trauma or a herniated disc. Research has shown that treatments utilizing stem cells have proven to be effective for both conditions. One study explored the use of autologous after undergoing hemilaminectomy, dogs with spontaneous spinal cord injuries from trauma showed significant enhancements in movement, pain perception, and sense of body position following treatment with BM-MSCs. A separate research study demonstrated a significant uptick in functional recuperation [370].

Dogs with acute disc herniation demonstrated positive results from MSC treatment, similar to dogs with traumatic spinal cord injuries. In cases of acute paraplegia, dogs treated with AD-MSCs epidurally regained their locomotion at a faster rate compared to dogs undergoing only surgical decompression. Conversely, the transplantation of autogenic BM-MSCs did not yield any significant improvement [438, 439].

Studies on the use of MSCs for treating traumatic spinal cord injury and disc herniation in dogs have shown encouraging results, but additional research is necessary to improve the recognized therapeutic benefits of MSC therapies. One potential method to achieve this enhancement is through tissue engineering. A study involving the incorporation of neural network tissue derived from canine MSCs into the spinal cord resulted in progressive improvement in motor function of the paralyzed limb.

Hence, additional research and advancements are essential to ascertain the efficacy of cell therapy and tissue bioengineering methods for treating spinal cord injuries has shown promise, particularly in cases of animals with naturally occurring damage, where the advancement of the condition differs substantially from those with experimentally induced pathologies. [440].

Kidneys

Chronic tubulointerstitial nephritis, tubular atrophy, and interstitial fibrosis are characteristic features of chronic kidney disease (CKD), a common medical condition observed in elderly cats. Kidney transplantation is currently the only treatment option that has the potential to restore renal function. As a result, stem cell-based therapies may present less invasive therapeutic alternatives. The preferred method of delivering stem cells is through intravenous injection, as intrarenal stem cell administration poses risks of serious side effects and anesthesia-related complications. Nevertheless, there have been no reported adverse effects associated with the intravenous delivery of allogeneic adipose-derived mesenchymal stem cells in cats with kidney disease, although there were no significant improvements in renal function observed in the short term. [441-443].

The utilization of MSC therapy in feline chronic glomerulonephritis syndrome (FCGS) has yielded exceedingly positive outcomes. Nevertheless, further investigation is imperative to determine The potential impact of different variables, including the origin of MSCs, frequency of treatment (one-time or repeated), and timing of application in correlation to the stage of the disease, on the efficacy of MSC therapy in cats suffering from CKD. Additionally, more extensive research is warranted to delve into the safety aspects of allogeneic cell therapy in felines, as there remains a dearth of studies in this particular domain.

Respiratory System

Respiratory conditions are frequently encountered within the field of veterinary medicine. Asthma, which encompasses various conditions Respiratory conditions in horses, such as recurrent airway obstruction (RAO) and inflammatory airway disease, present a notable medical obstacle that currently lacks a definitive remedy. Various factors including exposure to moldy hay, pollen, and dusty straw are implicated in the onset and progression of these conditions of this ailment. Common symptoms in affected horses include persistent coughing, increased effort to breathe at rest, and reduced tolerance for physical activity. Treatment options typically involve the use of corticosteroids, bronchodilators, or modifications to the animal's environment to alleviate clinical manifestations. Nevertheless, alternative therapeutic strategies are needed to mitigate potential adverse effects associated with these traditional medications. In cases of horses afflicted with RAO, novel approaches to treatment are imperative [373] investigated the impact of intratracheal injections of bone marrow-derived mononuclear cells (BM-MNCs) on the progression of respiratory inflammation. In contrast to oral therapy with dexamethasone and single intratracheal delivery of autogenic cells, BM-MNCs reduced the clinical symptoms and the inflammatory reaction in horses with RAO. After cell therapy, IL-10 levels rose and were noticeably greater than in the dexamethasone-treated control group. The findings of this investigation are consistent with those of experimental studies in dogs [374] and cats that used induced respiratory circumstances [444].

Eye

Ophthalmology is actively involved in researching the potential use of stem cell therapy. Certain eye disorders, like corneal ulcers, can be effectively treated using existing methods.

Following the treatment, all four animals exhibited significant improvements, characterized by restoration of the epithelial surface and reduction in inflammation levels. [445].

In another study, the administration of autologous BM-MSC via subconjunctival route resulted in improved immune-mediated keratitis in 75% of horses. This improvement was manifested by enhanced corneal clarity, decreased local neovascularization, and reduced surface irregularities. The immunomodulatory effects of MSCs appear to have a positive impact on equine recurrent uveitis (ERU), as evidenced by decreased IFN- production by CD4+ T cells isolated from horses with ERU following exposure to AD-MSCs in a laboratory setting. It has been established that signaling pathways involving PGE2 and cell-to-cell interactions contribute to the suppression of CD4+ T cell activation. [446].

The impressive results achieved through the subconjunctival implantation of allogeneic AD-MSCs, which led to the promising success of MSC therapy in treating conditions such as feline eosinophilic keratitis (FEK) has led to a notable decrease in clinical signs. Similarly, the effective treatment of keratoconjunctivitis sicca (KCS), also known as dry eye syndrome, in dogs using MSCs has been encouraging. A significant and lasting reduction in clinical symptoms was observed when allogeneic AD-MSCs were locally implanted around the lacrimal glands. [447, 448].

The evolution of stem cell research: an overview of historical milestones, current developments, and future prospects

Categorization of stem cells

Stem cells, residing within the human body, are a type of undifferentiated cells endowed with the remarkable capacity to differentiate into various cell types and undergo self-renewal. These cells can be found in both embryos and adult tissues, undergoing several stages of specialization. As cells progress through these stages, their developmental potency decreases, with unipotent stem cells having a limited capacity for differentiation compared to pluripotent stem cells. The classifications of stem cells are discussed in this chapter to provide a foundation for understanding subsequent chapters.

Totipotent stem cells possess the unique ability to divide and differentiate into all cell types within an organism, including both embryonic and extra-embryonic structures. A well-known example of a totipotent cell is the zygote, formed from the fusion of a sperm and egg, with the potential to develop into any cell within the three germ layers or contribute to placental formation. Following approximately four days of development, the inner cell mass of the blastocyst transitions into a pluripotent state, serving as a source of cells with broader potential.

Pluripotent stem cells possess the ability to differentiate into cells of all germ layers, excluding extraembryonic structures like the placenta. Embryonic stem cells, for instance, are one type of pluripotent stem cells that are obtained Stem cells obtained from the inner cell mass of preimplantation embryos represent one example of pluripotent cells. Another illustration is provided by induced pluripotent stem cells, which originate from the epiblast layer of embryos that have been implanted. These cells exhibit differing degrees of pluripotency, with some displaying high potency akin to embryonic stem cells and induced pluripotent stem cells, while others exhibit lower potency such as multipotent, oligopotent, or unipotent cells. The teratoma formation assay is one method used to evaluate their potential and range of differentiation capabilities. iPSCs, which are generated artificially from somatic cells, exhibit properties similar to PSCs and hold great promise for current and future applications in regenerative medicine.

Multipotent stem cells exhibit a more limited range of differentiation compared to pluripotent stem cells, yet they have the capacity to specialize into distinct cell types within specific lineages. For instance, haematopoietic stem cells have the ability to mature into various blood cell types. Following differentiation, a haematopoietic stem cell transitions into an oligopotent cell, with its differentiation potential confined to cells within its particular lineage. Nevertheless, certain multipotent cells have the ability to transform into different cell types outside their lineage, indicating a classification as pluripotent cells.

Oligopotent stem cells possess the capability to differentiate into multiple cell types. An example of this is a myeloid stem cell, which can give rise to white blood cells but not red blood cells.

Unipotent stem cells are defined by their restricted capacity for specialization and remarkable capability for continuous proliferation, making them a highly viable option for therapeutic use in the field of regenerative medicine. These particular cells possess the ability to produce only a singular type of cell, such as dermatocytes.

The science of stem cell research

The inner wall of this blastocyst harbors short-lived embryonic stem cells. Within blastocysts, there are two specific cell types: the inner cell mass (ICM) responsible for generating epiblasts and initiating fetus development, and the trophectoderm. Blastocysts play a critical role in regulating the microenvironment that surrounds the ICM.

The TE continues to mature and create necessary extraembryonic support structures vital for the successful commencement of embryo development, such as the placenta. As the TE focuses on building specialized support systems, the ICM cells retain their undifferentiated, fully pluripotent, and proliferative nature. [449].

The inherent ability of stem cells to differentiate into any cell type within an organism is known as pluripotency. Human embryonic stem cells, specifically derived from the inner cell mass (ICM), have the potential to form various cell types.

During the process of embryogenesis, cells undergo a process of organization into distinct germ layers known as endoderm, mesoderm, and ectoderm. These germ layers subsequently differentiate into various cells and tissues within the fetus, ultimately contributing to the development of the fully formed adult organism.

Following differentiation into a specific germ layer, human embryonic stem cells become multipotent stem cells, capable of giving rise to cells within that particular layer. This process is relatively brief within human development.

Once differentiated, pluripotent stem cells can be found throughout the organism as undifferentiated cells, exhibiting the crucial abilities of self-renewal through cell division and specialization into specific cell types based on specific physiological cues. [450].

Fig. 4

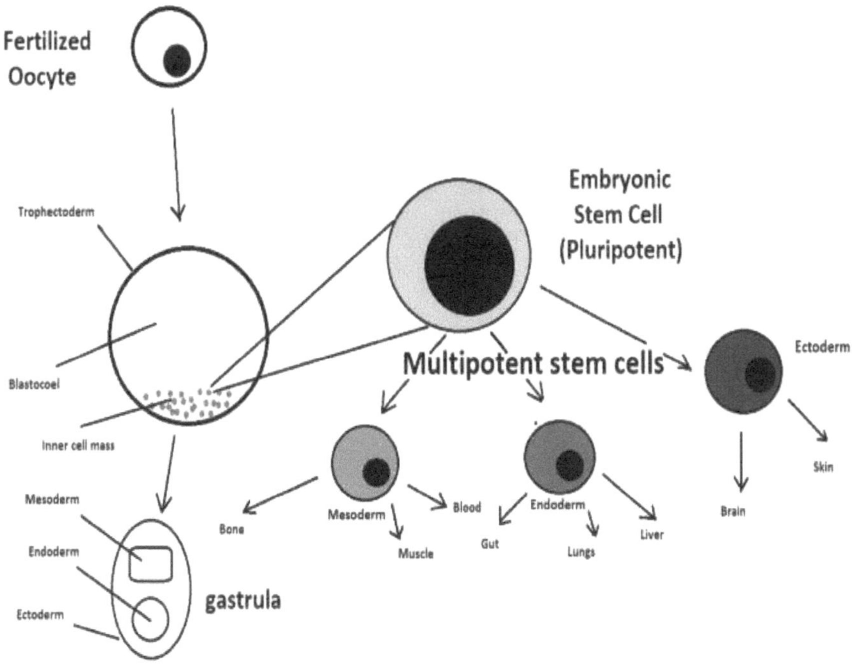

Oocyte maturation and stem cell development: The blastocoel, originating from oocytes, harbors pluripotent embryonic stem cells which later transform into mesodermal, ectodermal, or endodermal cells. The blastocoel progresses into the gastrula stage.

Factors influencing the differentiation of stem cells can be classified as either external, including physical cell interactions or chemical signals from nearby tissue, or internal, which are signals controlled by genes within the DNA

Stem cells serve as the body's internal repair mechanisms. The renewal and generation of new cells are continuous throughout an organism's lifespan. The activity of stem cells varies depending on the specific organ they inhabit; for instance, in the bone marrow, their proliferation is ongoing, while in organs like the pancreas, proliferation occurs only under specific physiological circumstances.

The process of stem cell differentiation into specialized cell types

The comprehensive development of the entire body

Throughout the process of division, the presence of various types of stem cells is contingent upon the developmental stage of the organism. Somatic stem cells, such as ESCs, can be identified during this stage. While it is feasible to derive ESCs without separating them from the TE, this combination does present limitations in terms of growth potential. Due to the restricted proliferative capabilities, it is typically advisable to avoid co-culturing these cells.

Embryonic stem cells (ESCs) are derived from the embryonic inner cell mass at approximately 4 days post-fertilization during the blastocyst stage of development. These cells are then cultivated in a dish with suitable culture medium. Sub-culturing the cells involves passage, a procedure commonly used for transferring cells to new dishes, although it may not be the most efficient method. The pluripotent nature of these cells is due to their ability to differentiate into any cell type within the organism.

Since the inception of research on ESCs, ethical concerns have surrounded their utilization in medical treatments. The majority of embryonic stem cells are derived from fertilized eggs obtained from in vitro fertilization procedures, rather than from naturally fertilized eggs in vivo.

Adult or somatic stem cells are undifferentiated cells that can be found throughout the body alongside specialized cells, post-development. These cells play a crucial role in facilitating the repair, growth, and replacement of cells lost on a daily basis. They have a limited ability to differentiate into various cell types, including the following categories: Mesenchymal stem cells are abundant in various tissues, with bone marrow serving as a source for cells that can differentiate into bone, cartilage, and fat cells. These stem cells exhibit pluripotent behavior, capable of potentially specializing in cells from any germ layer. Neural cells are responsible for the generation of nerve cells, as well as their supporting cells known as oligodendrocytes and astrocytes.

Haematopoietic stem cells contribute to the production of different blood cell types, including red blood cells, white blood cells, and platelets. Skin stem cells are responsible for generating keratinocytes, which form a protective layer on the skin.

The proliferation period of somatic stem cells is longer than that of Embryonic Stem Cells (ESCs), and these cells can be reprogrammed to return to a pluripotent state. This can be achieved by transferring an adult nucleus into an oocyte's cytoplasm or by fusing it with a pluripotent cell, a technique famously used in the cloning of Dolly the sheep.

Human Embryonic Stem Cells (hESCs) play a crucial role in the overall development of the body, with the ability to differentiate into various types of cells with different levels of potency such as pluripotent, multipotent, totipotent, and unipotent. (Fig. 5) [450].

Fig. 5

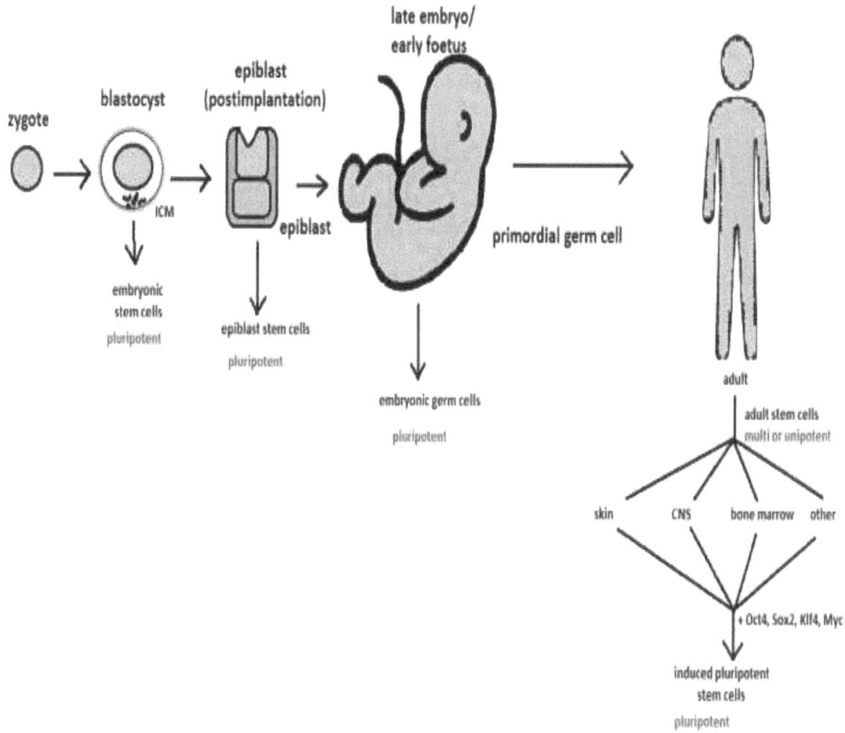

The process of stem cell potency changing throughout human body development is a complex and evolving phenomenon. It involves a range of cells starting from pluripotent cells in the blastocyst to unipotent cells in tissues such as the skin, central nervous system, or bone marrow. The capacity to transform cells back to a pluripotent state can be accomplished by generating induced pluripotent stem cells using crucial factors like Oct4, Sox2, Klf4, or the Myc gene.

Pluripotent cells possessing the ability to give rise to extraembryonic tissues are referred to as totipotent. Multipotent cells have limitations in their differentiation capabilities within a specific tissue. Stem cells responsible for generating a single lineage of cells within a tissue may be described as either oligo- or unipotent.

Quality assessment of induced pluripotent stem cells and their identification based on variations in morphology

To effectively incorporate iPSC lines for therapeutic purposes, it is essential to verify the consistency of stem cell lines derived from different individuals. Various critical quality control procedures encompass:

Analyzed through short tandem repeat analysis, which entails examining predetermined loci on the DNA samples to ascertain the precise quantity of repetitive units. Typically comprising 2 to 13 nucleotides repeated multiple times along the DNA strand, polymerase chain reaction is utilized to evaluate the lengths of these short tandem repeats. It is advisable to perform genotyping on the original tissue source, cells, as well as iPSC seed and master cell banks.

Identity analysis - Thorough examination is imperative in order to distinguish stem cell lines accurately to avoid unintended errors and the pollution of other lines.

Residual vector testing - It is crucial to conduct assessments to detect the presence of reprogramming vectors integrated into the host genome, as their emergence can present potential hazards. This testing method is frequently utilized for the creation of top-notch iPSC lines. The recognized standard for research-grade iPSC line collections of superior quality is ≤ 1 plasmid copies per 100 cells. Specific regions that are consistent across all plasmids, such as EBNA and CAG sequences, should be the focus during the evaluation process. [451].

In order to accurately represent the test responses, it is necessary to establish a standard curve using carrier gDNA from a well-characterized hPSC line. The inclusion of internal reference gDNA sequences is crucial for determining plasmid copies per cell, enabling the quantification of markers like RNaseP or hTERT.

The prolonged culture of hESCs may lead to the accumulation of culture-induced mutations, highlighting the importance of maintaining genomic integrity. Karyotype testing involves rejuvenating representative samples and culturing them for 48-72 hours before harvesting cells for karyotypic analysis. If any abnormalities are detected in the initial 20 karyotypes, it is essential to conduct a repeat analysis on a fresh sample. Persistent abnormalities lead to the classification of the line as abnormal, with recurrent deviations requiring thorough documentation.

While karyotyping is a critical quality control measure for stem cells, the SNP array discussed later in this text provides significantly higher resolution, approximately 50 times greater. [452].

In evaluating stem cell quality, it is imperative to conduct tests for harmful human adventitious agents such as hepatitis C or human immunodeficiency virus. This assessment is particularly crucial when non-xeno-free culture agents are used.

Bacteriology assessments for bacterial or fungal sterility are typically conducted using culture- or broth-based tests as recommended by the corresponding pharmacopoeia in the jurisdiction where the work is conducted.

Single nucleotide polymorphism arrays are a form of DNA microarray utilized to identify population variations and subchromosomal alterations, including copy-neutral loss of heterozygosity, to gain understanding into cell transformation. The SNP analysis entails labeling broken nucleic acid sequences with fluorescent dyes, using a grid with fixed allele-specific oligonucleotide (ASO) probes, and then recognizing, documenting, and analyzing the signals. [452].

Flow cytometry is a technique that utilizes light to quantify and describe cells in a diverse fluid mixture. This innovative method allows scientists to efficiently and precisely extract data from fluid mixtures containing viable cells. The cells are guided through a confined pathway, where specialized sensors detect the light emitted or bent by the cells upon exposure to illumination. Afterwards, the gathered information is scrutinized, categorized, and amalgamated to form a thorough examination of the specimen.

Phenotypic pluripotency assays are vital for identifying undifferentiated cells in the context of successful stem cell therapy. One defining characteristic of stem cells is their specific morphology, which includes a high ratio of nucleus to cytoplasm and a noticeable nucleolus. These cells typically exhibit a flat shape with distinct borders, distinguishing them from differentiating colonies that consist of loosely clustered cells with irregular boundaries. [452].

It is crucial to maintain images of both exemplary and subpar colonies for every cell line in laboratory settings in order to have a reference point for assessing culture quality when uncertainty arises. The creation of embryoid bodies or the controlled differentiation of monolayer cultures to generate cell types characteristic of the three embryonic germ layers is necessary. It should be emphasized that colonies grown under varying conditions may exhibit distinct morphologies. [454].

Histone modification and DNA methylation are mechanisms that can ensure quality control when assessing epigenetic status. During the differentiation of stem cells, DNA methylation can lead to the silencing of genes associated with pluripotency, limiting the potential for differentiation. Conversely, certain genes may undergo demethylation to become activated. It is crucial to highlight that the epigenetic profile of stem cells plays a significant role in determining their identity and morphology. Research by Brindley underscores the interconnectedness between epigenetic modifications, pluripotency, and the conditions in which cells expand, highlighting the importance of Serum-dependent unmethylated regions. [455- 458].

The process of obtaining human embryonic stem cells and the culture medium used for their maintenance

Various techniques can be utilized to generate hESCs, ranging from traditional culturing methods to sophisticated approaches like laser-assisted methodologies or microsurgery. It is imperative to precisely define the differentiation of hESCs in order to prevent the development of teratomas. (Fig. 6).

Fig. 6

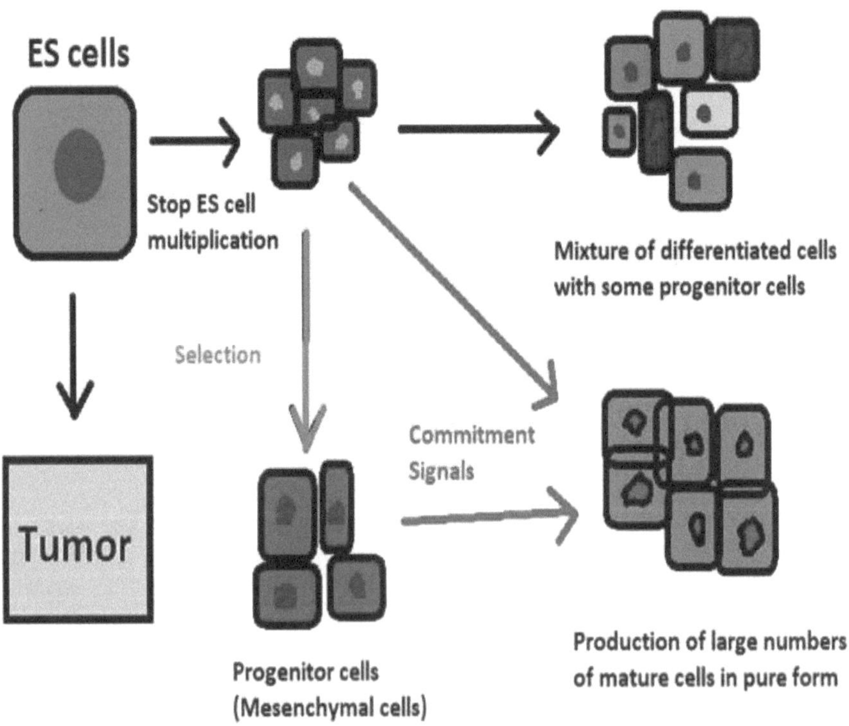

The natural progression of human embryonic stem cells leads to the creation of a diverse group of cells with varying characteristics. In contrast, the introduction of specific signals for cell differentiation, such as soluble factors and optimized culture conditions, allows for the identification and isolation of progenitor cells, leading to more controlled outcomes.

Human embryonic stem cells have the inherent ability to undergo spontaneous differentiation, resulting in the formation of embryonic bodies (EBs). These EBs provide a useful alternative to utilizing actual embryos or animals in studying their impact on early human development. Various techniques can be employed to generate EBs, including bioreactor culture, hanging drop culture, and microwell technology. Through these methodologies, distinct precursor cells can be effectively cultivated in a controlled laboratory setting. [460-463].

The crucial aspect of these cultivation techniques involves isolating the inner cell mass for the cultivation of future human embryonic stem cells (hESCs) as depicted in Figure 7. It is stressed that special care must be taken to control spontaneous differentiation. Once the cell colony reaches the appropriate size, the cells need to be separated. The presence of pluripotent cells typically lasts for 1-2 days. Due to ethical concerns surrounding the use of gastrulas in traditional hESC procedures, it has been discovered that hESCs can also be sourced from four-cell embryos, resulting in a higher likelihood of embryo survival. In their study, only growth-arrested cells from in vitro fertilization were utilized. [464- 468]

Fig. 7

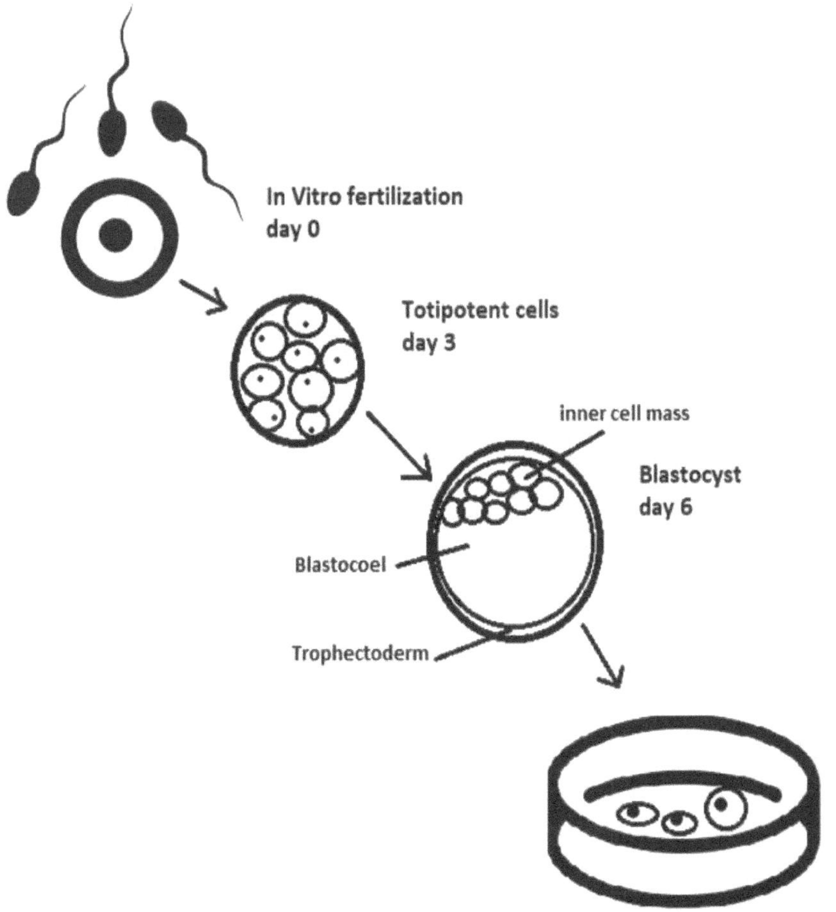

Pluripotent stem cells can be cultivated in a laboratory setting. Totipotent cells form three days post-fertilization, followed by the development of blastocysts containing inner cell mass (ICM) on the sixth day. The pluripotent stem cells derived from the ICM can be reliably transferred onto a culture dish.

Cell passaging is the act of generating smaller cell groupings on a new culture substrate. Several important passaging methods are employed during this procedure. Enzymatic dissociation is a technique which utilizes enzymes to disassemble proteins and adhesion sites that bind the cell colony.

This method is considered gentler compared to manual passaging. It is important to note that human embryonic stem cells (hESCs) should not be left alone after passaging as solitary cells are more susceptible to cell death. An example of an enzyme used in this process is collagenase type IV. [469- 471].

Contrastingly, manual passaging involves the utilization of cell scratchers, without the requirement for selecting specific cells. This step is typically conducted during the initial phases of deriving a cell line. [472].

The utilization of trypsin facilitates a seamless and efficient passage of healthy human embryonic stem cells (hESCs). GMP-quality recombinant trypsin is easily obtainable for this procedure. However, there is a potential disadvantage in terms of diminishing the pluripotency and viability of the stem cells. One method to address this concern is by employing a rho-associated protein kinase (ROCK) inhibitor to inhibit the use of trypsin. [472- 474].

EDTA functions by sequestering divalent cations, thereby indirectly inhibiting cellular adhesion and facilitating cell detachment [475].

Stem cells necessitate a combination of growth factors and nutrients for their differentiation and maturation. It is recommended to replace the medium on a daily basis.

Conventional techniques utilized for the cultivation of human embryonic stem cells (hESCs) involve the utilization of Research has demonstrated that when human embryonic stem cells (hESCs) are cultured with mouse embryonic fibroblasts (MEFs) as a supporting layer and bovine serum as the culture medium, they exhibit the presence of the non-human sialic acid, N-glycolylneuraminic acid (NeuGc). Additionally, the utilization of feeder layers in this culture system has been observed aids in controlling excessive cell proliferation with the incorporation of factors like leukaemia inhibitory factor (LIF). [476- 478].

The initial feeder layer-free culture technique may be enhanced by the addition of serum replacement and laminin [479], leading to the maintenance of stable karyotypes in stem cells and sustained pluripotency for a period exceeding one year.

The starting medium for culturing cells may consist of serum, such as foetal calf serum (FCS), Synthetic serum substitutes such as SSS, knockout serum replacement (KOSR), or StemPro are commonly used in cellular research. The essential components in the basic culture medium usually consist of DMEM/F12 medium, selenium, sodium bicarbonate, L-ascorbic acid, transferrin, insulin, TGFβ1, and FGF2. The compatibility of culture systems designed for hESCs with iPSC cultures without modification remains uncertain. [480].

Significant breakthrough in the field of stem cell therapy

In 2006, a notable advancement in the field of stem cell therapy took place when scientists Shinya Yamanaka and Kazutoshi Takahashi discovered the possibility of transforming multipotent adult stem cells into a pluripotent state without endangering the fetus. By utilizing retrovirus-mediated transduction to introduce four transcription factors primarily found in embryonic stem cells into mouse fibroblasts, they were able to prompt the fibroblasts to transform into pluripotent cells. (Fig. 8) [483].

A novel type of stem cells was designated as iPSCs. Following this breakthrough, the replication of this experiment with human cells proved successful. As a result, a new avenue in stem cell research was unveiled, yielding iPSC lines that are adaptable and compatible with specific patients. Recent research endeavors have shifted towards minimizing the risk of cancer development and enhancing the conduction system within these cells. [484]

Fig. 8

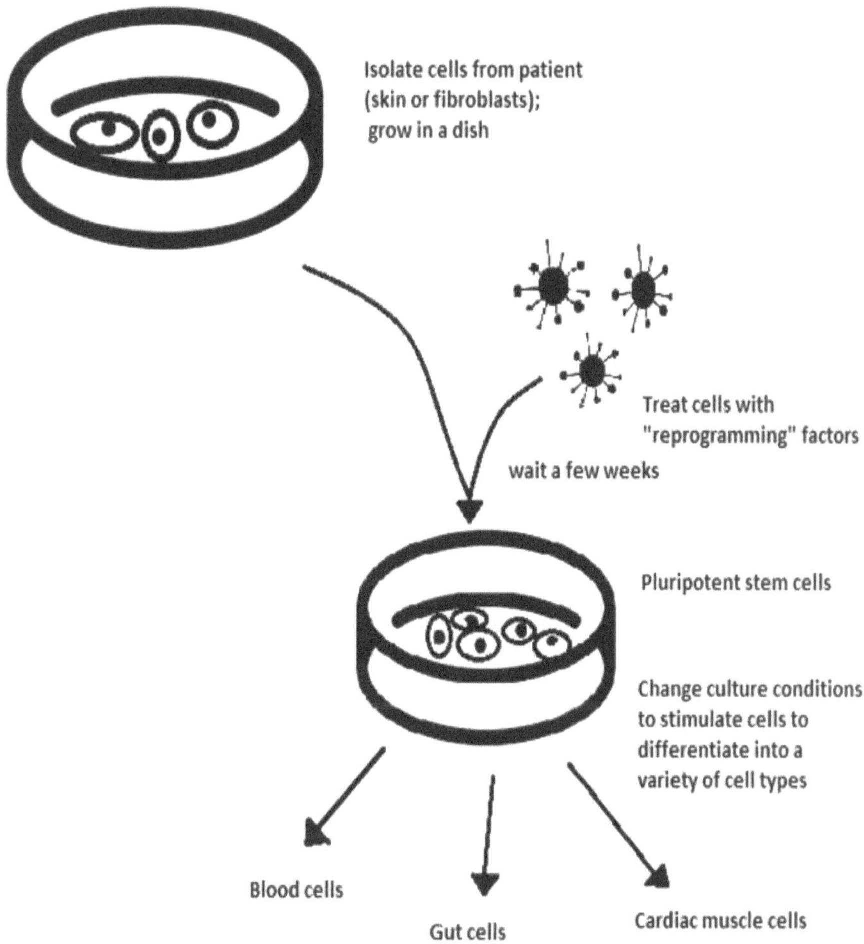

The induction of pluripotency in isolated patient somatic cells through retroviral-mediated transduction leads to a transformation where the target cells relinquish their somatic cell characteristics and regain pluripotency, allowing them to differentiate into various cell types within the human body.

The pivotal moment was shaped by previous breakthroughs that occurred in 1962 and 1987. The earlier breakthrough involved scientist John Gurdon achieving successful frog cloning by transferring a nucleus from a frog's somatic cells into an oocyte. His experiment yielded significant findings, challenging the existing belief that cell differentiation is irreversible and indicating the potential for somatic cells to regain pluripotency. [485, 486].

The latter discovery, by Davis R.L., centered on fibroblast DNA subtraction and identified three genes that had previously been present in myoblasts. The introduction of just one of these genes, referred to as myogenic differentiation 1 (Myod1), resulted in the transformation of fibroblasts into myoblasts. This demonstrates the potential for cell reprogramming and the ability to convert cells from one lineage to another. [487].

iPSCs, or induced pluripotent stem cells, are a type of cell that is generated by reprogramming adult cells to behave like embryonic stem cells

Pluripotency is a characteristic typically found only in embryonic stem cells, however, it is feasible to induce fully differentiated cells to regain this pluripotent state. The method of direct reprogramming involves the transformation of differentiated somatic cells into iPSC lines capable of developing into any cell type within an organism. This reprogramming process is centered around the activation of oncogenes like Myc and Klf4, leading to the downregulation of genes that promote genomic stability.

Furthermore, cell reprogramming implicates modifications in histones. These various processes have the potential to introduce mutagenic risks, eventually resulting in an elevated occurrence of mutations. Quinlan et al. stated that_different pathogens can be directly__binvolved in the infection processiątidak(tolua) [488]

Meticulous analysis was conducted on fully pluripotent mouse iPSCs utilizing advanced techniques for comprehensive whole-genome DNA sequencing and sophisticated algorithms designed for detecting structural variations (SV). The research findings confirmed the presence of isolated mutations in non-coding regions, but no retrotransposon insertions were identified in the iPSCs. Consequently, it was determined that existing reprogramming methodologies are capable of generating fully pluripotent iPSCs without significant genomic aberrations.

As pluripotent hESCs transition into specialized somatic cells during development, pivotal alterations occur in the epigenetic landscape of these cells. This process involves the regulation or facilitation of gene transcription specific to each cell type. When somatic cells are reprogrammed utilizing transcription factors, a complete reshaping of the epigenetic framework is necessary to yield iPSCs with pluripotent capabilities. Nevertheless, individual tissue cells undergo distinctive somatic genomic methylation, which impacts transcription and may lead to modifications in induced pluripotency. [489, 490].

Origin of induced pluripotent stem cells

Pluripotent cells have the ability to continuously proliferate and transform into various cell types, making them a valuable and limitless resource for tissue replacement in cases of injury or disease. Induced pluripotent stem cells (iPSCs) eliminate the necessity for embryos in stem cell treatments.

Initially, fibroblasts were utilized to generate iPSCs, requiring a biopsy for cell extraction. This prompted further exploration into more readily available cell sources. The inquiry uncovered the potential for utilizing readily obtainable cells like peripheral blood cells, keratinocytes, and renal epithelial cells derived from urine specimens.

A different method for stem cell treatment includes activating a patient's intrinsic stem cells to divide and differentiate, a natural occurrence seen in skin repair during wound healing. A notable breakthrough in 2008 exhibited the effective transformation of pancreatic exocrine cells into functioning beta cells that can create insulin. [491].

Fibroblasts are considered the most ideal source of stem cells, particularly due to their rapid and regulated stimulation, making them alluring from a logistical perspective. [492].

Assessment of teratoma formation

The regenerative medicine field is currently centered on exploring the self-renewal and differentiation capabilities of iPSCs, generating significant interest and attention. A crucial aspect of studying these capabilities involves conducting a quality-control test, with the teratoma formation assay being among the most essential. Teratomas, which are benign tumors, exhibit rapid in vivo growth and distinctively possess the capacity to differentiate into tissues from all three germ layers concurrently. Due to the remarkable pluripotency displayed by teratomas, this particular assay serves as a critical evaluation of iPSCs' capabilities. [493].

The rate of teratoma formation was found to be higher in human induced pluripotent stem cells (iPSCs) compared to human embryonic stem cells (hESCs). This discrepancy could be attributed to variations in differentiation methods and the source of the cells. Typically, the teratoma assay involves the subcutaneous or intratesticular/intrarenal injection of iPSCs into immunodeficient mice. Following injection, the formation of immature but discernible tissues such as kidney tubules, bone, cartilage, or neuroepithelium can be observed. The location of injection may influence the efficiency of teratoma formation. [494- 496].

In this assay, three distinct groups of markers are utilized to discern the cells originating from the germ layers.

Teratoma formation assays are widely recognized as the benchmark for proving the pluripotency of human induced pluripotent stem cells, demonstrating their adaptability in natural settings. These assays, by virtue of generating actual tissue formations, serve as valuable tools for delineating different cell lineages. [497, 498].

Differentiation under specific guidance

For stem cells to be successful in therapeutic uses, it is crucial that they are directed to develop into particular cell types on demand; otherwise, the potential of regenerative medicine could be compromised. The differentiation of embryonic stem cells is particularly critical due to the possible formation of teratomas in vivo if these cells remain in their undifferentiated state.

The comprehension and utilization of signaling pathways for differentiation play a vital role in achieving success in regenerative medicine. Directed differentiation involves the replication of signals that cells typically receive as they progress through various stages of development. [499].

The extracellular environment is a pivotal factor in influencing cellular behavior. Through careful manipulation of cultural conditions, one can steer differentiation pathways and cultivate cultures rich in particular precursors in a laboratory setting. Nonetheless, replicating this effect in a living organism poses challenges. Therefore, there is a pressing need to establish cultural conditions that facilitate uniform and improved differentiation of embryonic stem cells into functional and desired tissues.

Hwang et al. [500] emphasized the necessity of an optimal culture method for embryonic stem cells to ensure self-renewal, particularly in the context The field of cell and tissue therapy aims to develop a method that does not rely on feeder layers or animal components in culture. The use of feeder cells is deemed unsuitable for the sustained growth of the necessary large quantities of undifferentiated human embryonic stem cells for therapeutic applications.

Numerous protocols governing the process of directed differentiation focus on mimicking the intricate process of inner cell mass formation that occurs during gastrulation. Pluripotent stem cells transition into ectodermal, mesodermal, or endodermal progenitors as part of their development during this critical phase. The utilization of small molecules or growth factors is vital in inducing the differentiation of stem cells into distinct progenitor cells, ultimately leading to the generation of the intended cell type.

Various signal intensities and molecular families, including fibroblast growth factors (FGFs), the Wnt family, the transforming growth factor-β superfamily (TGFβ), and bone morphogenic proteins (BMP), can influence the formation of germ layers in vivo. [500-503].

Every potential factor must undergo testing at different concentrations and exposure times, as the exact timing and concentrations at which developing cells in embryos are impacted during differentiation remain uncertain. For example, molecular blockers of natural BMP and Wnt signaling have been utilized to aid in the formation of ectoderm from embryonic stem cells. On the other hand, temporary exposure to Wnt and lower levels of TGFβ family members stimulate the differentiation of mesodermal cells. In the case of endoderm development, a higher concentration of activin A may be necessary. [504- 507].

There are various established procedures regarding the techniques for generating precursor cells of each germ layer, including cardiomyocytes, hepatocytes, renal cells, lung cells, motor neurons, intestinal cells, and chondrocytes. [508- 515].

The deliberate induction of iPSCs or ESCs into specific cell types, such as hepatocytes, has the potential to advance our understanding of the molecular processes involved in human liver development. Furthermore, this process offers the opportunity to generate artificial hepatocytes for the purpose of conducting drug toxicity assessments. [516].

The levels of concentration and the length of activity of a specific signaling molecule can have an influence on numerous factors. Sadly, the current exorbitant price of recombinant factors is anticipated to limit their extensive use in the medical field. An alternative and more beneficial method involves utilizing small molecules, which have the ability to efficiently adjust specific signaling pathways by either activating or deactivating them.

These small molecules improve the efficiency of reprogramming, leading to cells that are better suited for the desired tissue type. This approach is not only cost-efficient but also prevents the activation of an immune response.

Successful instances of small-molecule cell therapies can be observed in the form of antagonists and agonists that target the Hedgehog pathway, which have demonstrated significant efficacy in motor neuron regeneration. [517].

Endogenous small molecules that play a role in embryonic development can also be utilized in vitro to stimulate cell differentiation. One such example is retinoic acid, known for its role in shaping the nervous system during development, which unexpectedly prompted the formation of retinal cells in human embryonic stem cells within a laboratory setting. [518, 519].

The success of differentiation factors depends on the functional maturity, efficiency, and proper introduction of the cells they produce to their in vivo counterparts. Various factors, including topography, shear stress, and substrate rigidity, are crucial in influencing the phenotype of these cells. [520].

The regulation of both biophysical and biochemical cues, alongside meticulous oversight of the biophysical setting and strategic management of hESC differentiation are critical components in ensuring optimal cultivation of stem cells.

The utilization of stem cells, along with their quality control for manufacturing processes and cultivation methods

Previous protocols for stem cell transplantation involved the use of animal-derived products, leading to concerns about the introduction of animal antigens or pathogens and necessitating a revision of the technique. As a result, the use of xeno-free alternatives is now considered essential when creating cell lines from fresh embryos and culturing them with human feeder cell lines. It is imperative in this process to substitute any non-human materials with xeno-free alternatives. [521- 525].

Utilization of stem cells in the field of medicine

Stem cells possess significant potential to emerge as a pivotal component of the field of medicine. Not only do they play a crucial role in the advancement of regenerative medicine, but studying them also provides valuable insights into the intricate processes involved in human development.

The differentiation between a stem cell and a specialized cell can be determined by examining the organization of their DNA. In stem cells, the DNA is intricately arranged with genes that are actively expressing. External signals trigger the start of the differentiation process, leading to the deactivation of unnecessary genes and the maintenance of essential ones for the cell's specific function. This process of gene regulation is reversible, and the potential for pluripotency can be achieved through genetic interactions. Research conducted by Takahashi and Yamanaka has provided valuable insights into this mechanism.

[526] as well as Loh et al. [527] have identified Oct3/4, Sox2, and Nanog as core transcription factors crucial for maintaining pluripotency, with Oct3/4 and Sox2 being particularly vital for the generation of induced pluripotent stem cells.

Numerous significant medical conditions, such as birth defects and cancer, can be attributed to issues with cell division and differentiation. At present, a variety of stem cell therapies exist for conditions like spinal cord injury, heart failure, retinal and macular degeneration, tendon ruptures, and type 1 diabetes. Research in the field of stem cells has the potential to enhance our comprehension of stem cell physiology, leading to the discovery of novel treatment methods for diseases that are presently untreatable. [528-530]

Transplantation of haematopoietic stem cells

For more than fifty years, haematopoietic stem cells have been the subject of extensive research, rendering them the most thoroughly studied tissue-specific stem cells. These cells provide a valuable model for the study of tissue-specific stem cells and show potential for use in regenerative medicine. [531]

Nevertheless, there are notable limitations to traditional sources of hematopoietic stem cells that must be acknowledged. Firstly, there exists a finite number of transplantable cells, and there is still a need to develop a more efficient method of collection.

Additionally, the challenge of identifying a compatible antigen-matched donor for transplantation poses difficulties, along with concerns related to viral contamination and immunoreactions that can compromise the effectiveness of conventional hematopoietic stem cell transplants. Given the multifaceted nature and potential risks associated with hematopoietic transplantation, it is typically reserved for patients with life-threatening conditions.

The application of induced pluripotent stem cells is essential in this procedure. Using a patient's own nonspecialized somatic cells as a source of stem cells ensures high immunological compatibility and greatly improves the chances of success.

Exploring the use of stem cells in pharmacological experimentation

Stem cells have the potential to be utilized in novel drug testing methodologies. By utilizing specific differentiated cells derived from pluripotent cells, experiments on living tissue can be conducted with a high degree of safety. Any adverse reactions can prompt adjustments to the drug formulations until an optimal level of efficacy is achieved.

This approach allows for the introduction of new drugs into the pharmaceutical market without subjecting live test subjects to any harm. Nonetheless, in order to accurately compare the effects of different drugs, it is imperative that testing conditions remain consistent. To this end, researchers must master the differentiation process to yield homogenous populations of differentiated cells.

Utilizing stem cells as an alternative to arthroplasty

One of the primary concerns for professional athletes is the potential for sustaining an injury, as it can frequently result in the premature conclusion of their athletic careers. This is particularly true in the case of tendon injuries, as the existing treatment approaches of conservative or surgical methods often yield suboptimal results. The issue with tendon injuries often stems from their inability to regenerate effectively. [532].

Moreover, in addition to tendon-related issues, there is a significant possibility of developing a pathological condition in the joints called osteoarthritis (OA). OA is widespread due to inadequate blood supply to the articular cartilage and its limited capacity for regeneration. While arthroplasty is a frequently used treatment for OA, it may not be suitable for younger patients who could outlive the implant, leading to the need for multiple future surgeries. Stem cell therapy could play a crucial role in preventing the onset of OA in such cases. Nevertheless, these procedures are still in the nascent stages of development, and further research is required for the long-term preservation of hyaline cartilage. [533, 534]

Osteonecrosis of the femoral head (ONFH) is a difficult medical condition characterized by the deterioration of the femoral head and the potential need for hip replacement surgery in younger individuals. While total hip arthroplasty (THA) is an effective treatment, it may not be the most suitable option for younger patients due to the prosthesis's limited lifespan. Numerous clinical studies have explored using stem cells as a treatment for ONFH, with many showing promising results such as decreased pain, enhanced mobility, and potentially avoiding the need for hip replacement surgery. [536-539].

Cell programming for rejuvenation

Ageing is a process that can be reversed at the epigenetic level. The first study on cell rejuvenation was published in 2011. It has been observed that cells taken from older individuals exhibit unique transcriptional patterns, - Elevated levels of oxidative stress, impaired mitochondria, and reduced telomere length are observed in aged cells as compared to younger cells. A theory suggests that the epigenetic age of adult somatic cells can be reset to zero when they are reprogrammed into induced pluripotent stem cells (iPSCs) in humans or mice. This hypothesis is rooted in an epigenetic model that suggests during fertilization, all signs of parental aging are eliminated from the zygote's genetic code and its aging process is restarted from the beginning. [540- 543].

Their research demonstrated the potential of these genes for effective regenerative therapies. One of the primary challenges faced in their approach was the necessity to develop a method that does not involve transgenic animals and does not require prolonged application.

The initial clinical implementation would likely focus on preventive measures aimed at halting or slowing the aging process. Subsequently, efforts could be made towards progressively rejuvenating elderly individuals. Potential ethical dilemmas, such as concerns related to overpopulation and its impact on the availability of food and energy, may arise as this method is further developed.[544, 545]

At present, it is crucial to understand the implementation of cell reprogramming technology in elderly animals and humans that do not have genetic modifications to eliminate signs of aging while preserving the epigenetic markers of cell differentiation.

Regenerative medicine approaches utilizing cell-based therapies

Stem cells have the capability to differentiate into a specific cell type necessary for the restoration of injured or compromised tissues. In situations where the demand for transplantable tissues and organs surpasses the availability, stem cells present a viable solution to the dilemma. Conditions such as macular degenerations, strokes, osteoarthritis, neurodegenerative diseases, and diabetes have shown significant improvements through this form of therapy. Through this innovative approach, it may be feasible to cultivate healthy cardiac muscle cells for subsequent transplantation into individuals with heart ailments. [98-100]

Fig. 9

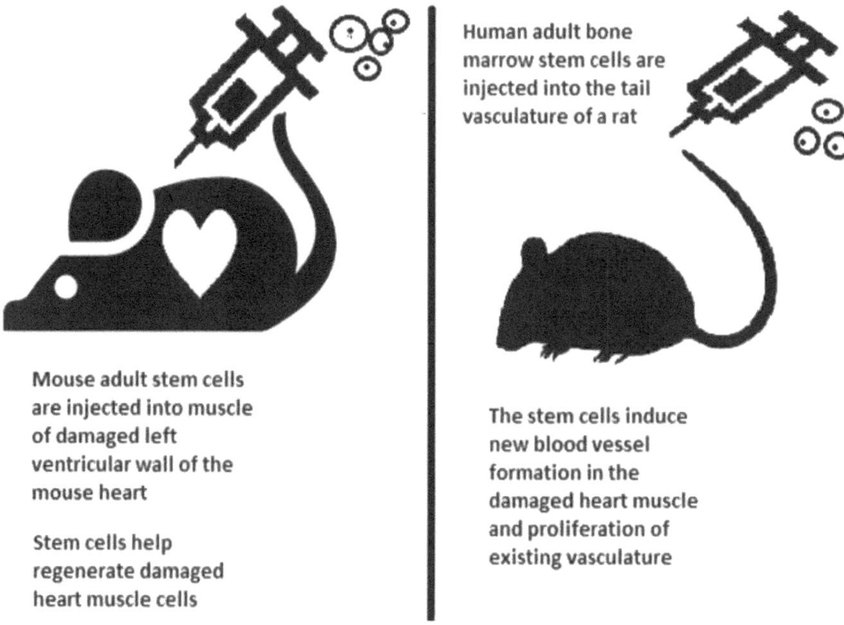

Experiments involving stem cells conducted on animals have demonstrated the essential role of stem cells in the advancement of regenerative medicine.

Type 1 diabetes is characterized by the destruction of insulin-producing cells in the pancreas as a result of an autoimmune response. Instead of relying on transplantation therapy, there is potential for stem cells to be directed towards developing into insulin-producing cells. [549].

Cellular stem resources and repositories for biological tissues

iPS cells possess an innate ability for both unlimited proliferation and specialization, making them highly appealing for present and future scientific pursuits. These cells can be preserved in a tissue bank to serve as a vital reservoir of human tissue for medical research. Unlike conventional differentiated tissue cells kept in laboratory conditions, iPS cells do not experience a decrease in their propagation abilities over time.

The umbilical cord is recognized for its abundance of mesenchymal stem cells, which can be cryopreserved immediately after birth for future use in therapies aimed at preventing potentially life-threatening illnesses in patients.

Stem cells derived from human exfoliated deciduous teeth, obtained from shed baby teeth, possess the capability to transform into a broader array of bodily tissues when compared to alternative forms of stem cells. [550]

- The procedures for collecting, isolating, and preserving SHED cells are straightforward and minimally invasive. Some of the benefits of storing these cells include ensuring a perfect match for transplantation as well as preventing immune reactions and cell rejection. [551]

- Easily manageable and comfortable for both the child and parent.
- Costs less than one-third of the expenses associated with storing cord blood.
- Does not raise the same ethical dilemmas as embryonic stem cells. [552]

- SHED cells possess the ability to differentiate into various types of solid tissues like neural, connective, dental, and bone tissue, unlike cord blood stem cells.
- SHED cells hold promise for benefiting close family members of the donor

Fertility diseases

In a study conducted in 2011 by Katsuhiko Hayashi and fellow researchers, the potential for creating sperm from induced pluripotent stem cells in mice was successfully demonstrated. The investigators were able to breed healthy and fertile offspring from infertile mice, achieving similar success in female mice where iPSCs produced fully functional eggs.

Individuals, who are at a higher likelihood of experiencing advantages from the preservation and transplantation of testicular tissue, particularly cancer patients, are those who are confronted with the potential loss of their spermatogonial stem cells (SSC). Well-established techniques for freezing both adult and pre-pubertal testicular tissue have been developed, showcasing their efficiency. [555, 556].

Qiuwan et al. [557] presented significant findings indicating that transplantation of human amniotic epithelial cells (hAEC) has the potential One potential method for improving ovarian function in mice involves inhibiting cell apoptosis and reducing inflammation in compromised ovarian tissue.

This approach holds potential for the treatment of premature ovarian failure or insufficiency in female cancer survivors.

Advancements in fertility treatments for humans are on the horizon, but there are multiple obstacles that need to be addressed. The primary challenge is ensuring that the process is highly effective, followed by the need to minimize the likelihood of tumor formation instead of the production of viable eggs or sperm.

Another hurdle to overcome is the development of techniques for maturing human sperm and eggs in a laboratory setting without the need for in vivo transplantation, which could pose risks of tumorigenesis or invasive procedures.

Treatment for untreatable neurodegenerative disorders

Stem cell therapy has shown substantial effectiveness in treating incurable neurodegenerative conditions like Parkinson's disease, Alzheimer's disease, and Huntington's disease.

It not only helps slow down the progression of these ailments but also addresses the root cause of the issue. The field of neuroscience has been revolutionized by the identification of neural stem cells (NSCs), challenging the belief that the adult central nervous system (CNS) lacked the ability to generate new neurons. [558, 559].

Neural stem cells have demonstrated the potential to enhance cognitive function in preclinical studies involving rodent models of Alzheimer's Disease. In their research, Awe et al. have successfully derived human induced pluripotent stem cells (iPSCs) from skin biopsy samples for the purpose of developing a neural stem cell-based therapy for Alzheimer's Disease.[560-563]

Degeneration of neurons in Parkinson's disease is localized, and human embryonic stem cells have the capability to effectively produce dopaminergic neurons. Parkinson's disease presents a promising opportunity for utilizing induced pluripotent stem cells for cell therapy. Despite its potential, this type of therapy is currently undergoing experimental research. Previously, aborted fetal brain tissue was utilized for treating patients with Parkinson's disease. While the outcomes varied, it demonstrated that treatments using pure stem cells hold significant promise as a viable therapy option. **[564, 565]**

The utilization of stem cells in the field of dentistry

Teeth pose a significant challenge for regenerative medicine due to their intricate structure and essential functions in articulation, mastication, and aesthetic appeal. Stem cells hold promise as a superior alternative to synthetic materials, with teeth being a natural and minimally invasive source of these cells.[566]

In the absence of stem cells, current periodontal treatments primarily involve growth factors, grafts, or surgery. Stem cells located in the periodontal ligament possess the ability to transform into osteoblasts or cementoblasts, and have also demonstrated versatility in differentiating into neural cells. The field of tissue engineering has proven to be effective in treating periodontal diseases, utilizing stem cells from the root apical regions to regenerate the periodontal ligament. The use of gene therapy involving adenoviruses carrying growth factors shows promise as a technique for tissue engineering in the field of periodontology. [567- 569]

Animal studies have demonstrated the effectiveness of dentin regeneration, leading to the formation of dentin bridges. [570].

Enamel regeneration is a more complex process compared to dentin regeneration. Once ameloblastoma cells differentiate into enamel, they are effectively eliminated, making restoration of enamel impossible. Research in the medical field has achieved the differentiation of bone marrow stem cells into ameloblastoma. [571].

Healthy dental tissue contains a significant quantity of regular stem cells, with a decrease in number occurring when the tissue undergoes trauma or inflammation. Various groups of dental stem cells can be identified and isolated. (Fig. 10) [572].

Fig. 10

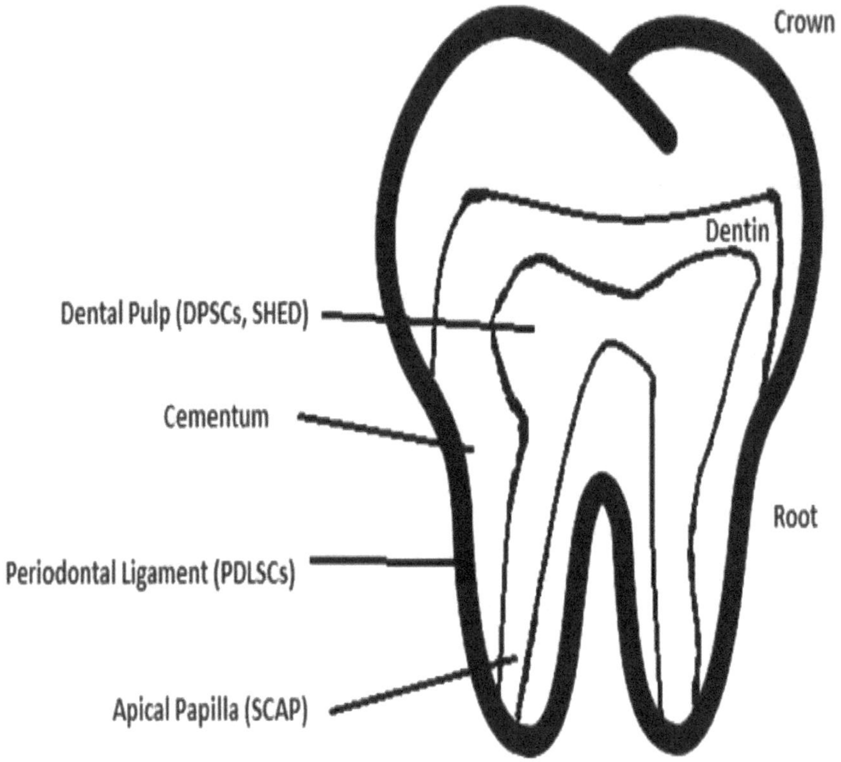

The phenomenon of stem cell localization in dental tissues has been extensively studied and documented. In particular, it has been observed that dental pulp stem cells (DPSCs) and human deciduous teeth stem cells (SHED) are present within the dental pulp, while periodontal ligament stem cells reside in the periodontal ligament. Furthermore, stem cells known as apical papilla stem cells (SCAP) are found in the apical papilla.

Dental pulp stem cells (DPSCs) are a type of stem cell found in the dental pulp

The initial discovery of dental stem cells from the human dental pulp occurred within the dental pulp itself. These particular stem cells demonstrate potential for bone and cartilage formation. (MSCs) are known for their high clonogenic ability upon isolation, with similar properties found in MSCs from adult tissues like bone marrow and adipose tissue, as well as from fetal tissues like the umbilical cord. These versatile cells display a strong capacity for differentiation. [573- 575].

Mesenchymal stem cells have the ability to transform into cells resembling odontoblasts and osteoblasts, which are responsible for the formation of dentin and bone. The most optimal locations for sourcing these cells are the third molars.

These cells have the potential to be utilized in a range of reconstructive procedures in maxillofacial and orthopaedic surgeries, extending beyond the confines of the oral cavity. Additionally, dental pulp stem cells exhibit the capability to generate all structures present in a fully developed tooth. [576].

Use of dental pulp stem cells can be enhanced by combining them with innovative therapies like periodontal tissue photobiomodulation. This technique, involving laser stimulation, is highly effective in promoting cell proliferation and differentiation into specific cell types. [577]. DPSCs can be induced to form neural cells to help treat neurological deficits.

The stem cells derived from human exfoliated deciduous teeth, known as SHED, exhibit a heightened rate of proliferation compared to dental pulp stem cells (DPSCs), and have the capacity to differentiate into diverse cell types, including neural cells, in addition to other mesenchymal and non-mesenchymal stem cell lineages. However, a notable limitation of SHED is their inability to form a complete dentin/pulp-like structure in vivo. Unlike embryonic stem cells, the use of SHED does not raise the same ethical concerns. Both DPSCs and SHED have demonstrated the ability to generate bone-like tissues in vivo, allowing for their potential application in periodontal, dentin, or pulp regeneration therapies. Additionally, DPSCs and SHED have shown promise in treating conditions such as neural deficits. DPSCs have been specifically evaluated and effectively utilized for reconstructing alveolar bone and mandibular defects. [578-581].

Periodontal ligament stem cells, commonly referred to as PDLSCs, are a type of stem cell found in the periodontal ligament

These cells are essential in the process of regenerating periodontal ligament or cementum tissue. They have the ability to transform into various types of mesenchymal cells that are involved in the production of collagen, adipocytes, cementum tissue, Sharpey's fibers, and osteoblast-like cells in a controlled setting. PDLSCs are present on the surfaces of both the root and alveolar bone, but they show greater potential for differentiation on the latter surface than the former. Due to their safety and effectiveness, PDLSCs have emerged as the primary choice for periodontal regeneration therapy [582- 584].

Stem cells derived from the apical papilla, known by the acronym SCAP

The cells being discussed are mesenchymal entities found within emerging root structures. These cells originate from the undeveloped permanent apical papilla in humans. SCAP are responsible for producing odontoblasts and play a significant role in apexogenesis. [585, 586].

Dental follicle stem cells, commonly referred to as DFCs, are a type of specialized cells found in the dental follicle region

The cells in question are a form of loose connective tissue that envelop the developing tooth germ. DFCs, or dental follicle cells, possess the ability to differentiate into cementoblasts, osteoblasts, and periodontal ligament cells. Additionally, they have exhibited notable proliferative capabilities even after undergoing more than 30 passages.

Harvested typically from the sac of a third molar, DFCs can be combined with a treated dentin matrix to create a tissue that resembles a root, complete with a pulp-dentin complex that facilitates the development of tooth roots. When stimulated by Hertwig's epithelial root sheath cells, DFC sheets can generate periodontal tissue, highlighting their potential as a highly promising material for tooth regeneration. [587- 590].

Regeneration of pulp tissue within the field of endodontics

Dental pulp stem cells have the ability to transform into odontoblasts. Limited techniques exist for the revitalization of the dental pulp. The initial approach involves an ex vivo procedure, where appropriate stem cells are cultivated on a scaffold and subsequently inserted into the root canal. [591].

The following method utilizes in vivo procedures, where stem cells are implanted into disinfected root canals after the formation of an in vivo apex. The use of a scaffold is crucial to prevent the movement of cells to surrounding tissues. Currently, only structures similar to pulp have been successfully produced.

Methods for inserting stem cells into the root canal can include the utilization of soft scaffolding or the application of stem cells during apexogenesis or apexification. Immature teeth are considered the most advantageous source for this procedure. The regeneration of nerve and blood vessel networks is crucial for the maintenance of healthy pulp tissue. [592, 593]

The primary focus of dental stem cells lies in the restoration of damaged dentin and pulp, as well as the repair of perforations. In the future, there is potential for the creation of entire teeth, which could revolutionize the field and diminish the need for implant procedures. Addressing mandibular and maxillary defects poses a significant challenge for dental stem cell research.

Gathering non-dental tissue cells through the process of dental stem cell differentiation

In 2013, a report indicated the feasibility of cultivating teeth from stem cells sourced externally, such as from urine. Tooth-like formations were induced and developed from pluripotent stem cells derived from human urine. While the physical traits of these structures closely resembled natural teeth, there was a slight deviation in terms of hardness. Despite this, the method shows great promise due to its non-invasive nature, affordability, and the ability to utilize somatic cells instead of embryonic ones. Additionally, the utilization of urine-derived stem cells did not result in tumor formation, and the use of autologous cells helps reduce the likelihood of rejection. [594-595].

Utilization of graphene in regenerative medicine utilizing stem cells is being explored

In recent years, there has been a growing trend in utilizing graphene and its derivatives as scaffold materials for facilitating the growth and differentiation of stem cells. Graphene and graphene oxide (GO) are known for their significant in-plane stiffness. Due to its carbon and aromatic network, graphene can interact with biomolecules either through covalent or non-covalent bonds, and its superior mechanical properties allow for a wide range of chemical modifications. The biocompatibility of graphene supports proper adhesion of cells, and it has shown promising results in promoting the proliferation and differentiation of stem cells. [596, 597].

Following successful experiments, graphene has demonstrated significant promise as a framework and directive for targeted stem cell differentiation. Utilization of graphene in the transplantation of hMSCs has proven effective in directing their specialization into specific cell types. Research has also delved into the enhancement of differentiation and proliferation rates facilitated by graphene. Graphene has been identified as a surface that enhances the attachment of growth factors and differentiation agents. [598].

Exploring the therapeutic efficacy of treatments utilizing extracellular vesicles

Extracellular vesicles (EVs) are produced by nearly all cells within an organism, including stem cells, and play a crucial role in intercellular communication by transporting their mRNAs, lipids, and proteins. Research by Oh et al. [599] illustrates that stem cells, in conjunction with their paracrine factors known as exosomes, have the potential to serve as therapeutic agents in addressing conditions such as skin aging. Exosomes, which are small membrane vesicles typically measuring 30–120 nm in diameter, are released by a variety of cell types.

lncRNAs possess the capacity to bind to particular loci and produce epigenetic regulators, leading to modifications in the epigenetic profile of recipient cells.

This unique characteristic suggests that exosomes may have a role in intercellular communication and the development of diseases such as cancer.

Numerous research studies have emphasized the potential therapeutic advantages of stem cell-derived exosomes in addressing conditions such as skin damage, renal, or pulmonary injuries. [599- 604].

In the process of skin aging, exposure to UV light, also known as "photoaging", is identified as the most significant factor. This exposure leads to extrinsic damage to the skin, resulting in addition to dryness, roughness, uneven pigmentation, blemishes, and the risk of skin cancer, extrinsic skin aging also manifests as a decrease in elasticity. In contrast, intrinsic skin aging is marked by a decline in the skin's ability to bounce back. Fibroblasts located in the skin dermis are tasked with producing key structural components such as procollagen and elastin fibers. These components act as building blocks of the skin's extracellular matrix or contribute significantly to tissue flexibility.

As individuals age, the efficiency and abundance of fibroblasts decrease, impacting skin health. [605, 606].

Stem cells have the ability to enhance the growth of dermal fibroblasts through the release of cytokines like platelet-derived growth factor (PDGF), transforming growth factor β (TGF-β), and basic fibroblast growth factor. According to research by Huh et al. [607], the use of a medium derived from human amniotic fluid stem cells (hAFSC) had a positive impact on skin rejuvenation following exposure to longwave UV radiation (UVA, 315-400 nm) by boosting the proliferation and migration of dermal fibroblasts. Furthermore, it was observed that apart from stimulating fibroblast function, hAFSC transplantation also led to advancements in treating conditions such as renal disorders, certain types of cancer, and stroke. [607-609].

The use of induced pluripotent stem cell-conditioned medium (iPSC-CM) lacking any animal-derived ingredients was found to promote the proliferation and migration of dermal fibroblasts. The process of natural cutaneous wound healing consists of three distinct phases: haemostasis/inflammation, proliferation, and remodelling. It is during the pivotal proliferation phase that fibroblasts migrate and multiply, highlighting its essential role in skin regeneration. Substances like iPSC-CM that influence this phase have the potential to enhance the overall healing process of cutaneous wounds. Furthermore, the paracrine actions carried out by iPSCs play a significant role in this therapeutic impact. [610-614].

The effects of extracellular vesicles (EVs) derived from human embryonic stem cells (hESCs) on in vitro cultured retinal glial progenitor Müller cells were investigated. These Müller cells have the ability to differentiate into retinal neurons.

The EVs were found to vary in size and were able to be taken up by the Müller cells, with their proteins playing a role in the initiation and maintenance of stem cell pluripotency. These vesicles from stem cells were responsible for inducing the trans-differentiation of cultured Müller cells into neurons. It is important to note, however, that this process was only conducted on retina acquired in vitro. There are several challenges associated with stem cell therapy.[612-614]

Despite the promising potential of stem cells in the field of medicine, there remain several challenges that must be addressed moving forward. The first and foremost concern pertains to ethics. The primary type of pluripotent stem cells, known as ESCs, have been at the center of ethical dilemmas since their discovery.

Initial therapies involving ESCs stirred controversy due to the ethical implications of extracting these cells from human embryos. The breakthrough in 1998, which revealed the ability to isolate ESCs, sparked hope for the treatment of various diseases, some of which were previously deemed incurable. However, the process of isolating ESCs resulted in the destruction of the embryo, which carried the potential for human life.Recognizing the significant potential of stem cell therapy, researchers have directed their efforts towards developing methods to isolate stem cells without compromising the source—the embryo. **Fig. 11**

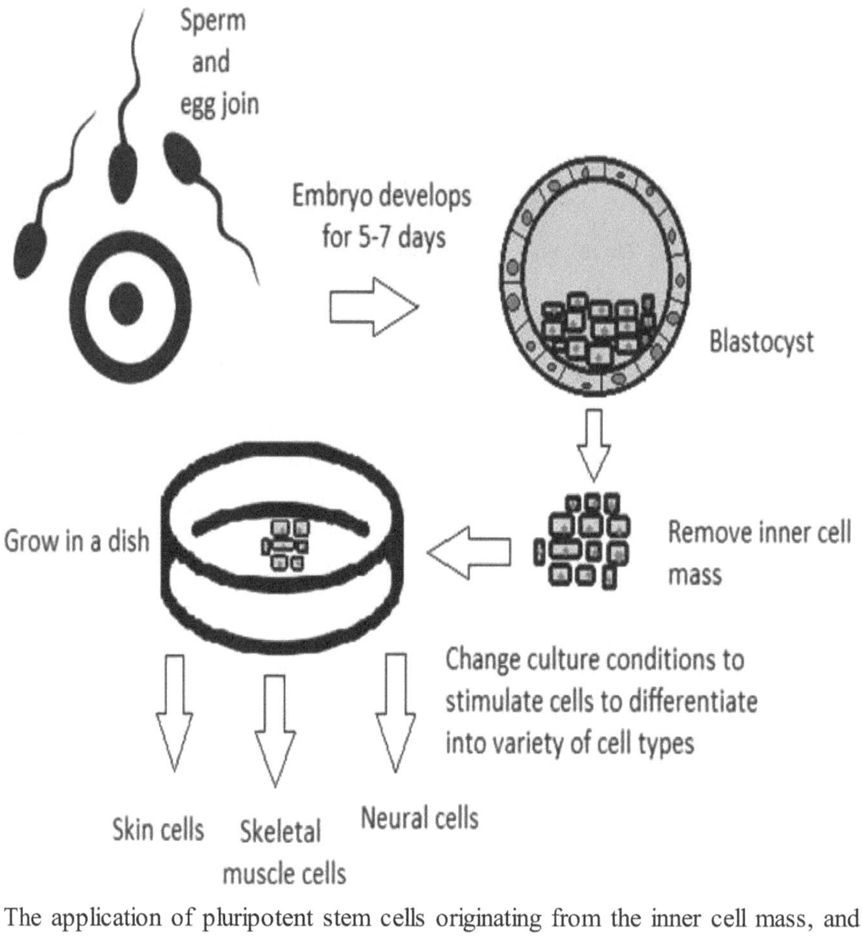

The application of pluripotent stem cells originating from the inner cell mass, and guiding their differentiation into particular cell types

Currently, human embryonic stem cells (hESCs) remain a subject of ethical debate as a potential source of cells for therapeutic purposes in tissue regeneration. The intricate control systems governing stem cells necessitate further exploration through in vitro observations. To ensure widespread acceptance, an evaluation of tumor risk is imperative for the utilization of stem cells in medical procedures. Establishing effective immunological tolerance between stem cells and the recipient's body poses another challenge. A promising approach involves deriving pluripotent cells from the patient's own tissues.

The newly generated cells must possess the capacity to fully substitute damaged or dysfunctional natural cells. Efforts are also underway to acquire stem cells without causing harm or discomfort to the patient or the donor. It is crucial to evaluate the controlled proliferation and differentiation of cells following transplantation to mitigate risks associated with regenerative procedures on human subjects. [615].

Limiting the utilization of iPSCs is the concern surrounding their potential to induce tumorigenesis. During the process of cellular reprogramming, there is a possibility that the expression of oncogenes could be upregulated. A technique was developed in 2008 to address this issue by allowing for the removal of oncogenes post achieving pluripotency, yet this method is still considered inefficient and time-consuming.

Enhancing the reprogramming process could involve the deletion of the tumor suppressor gene p53, however, this gene also plays a crucial role in cancer regulation, making its elimination to prevent further mutations in reprogrammed cells unfeasible. The efficacy of the process has been a concern, but it has shown improvement over time. [616].

Challenges pertaining to stem cells that may arise in the future

Scientific and medical advancements that pave the way in new territory must be vigilantly monitored to ensure they adhere to ethical standards and are safe. Stem cell therapy, due to its significant impact on various aspects of life, should be subject to the same oversight.

There are numerous challenges surrounding stem cells, with a primary concern being the imperative need to thoroughly comprehend the mechanisms by which stem cells operate in animal models as a first step. This critical stage cannot be bypassed, as fear of the unknown remains the primary obstacle to the widespread acceptance of this procedure.

Improving the effectiveness of controlling the direction of stem cell differentiation is crucial in order to enhance the dependability and credibility of stem cells for everyday patients. Furthermore, the extensive nature of the process poses a significant obstacle, especially in relation to potential upcoming stem cell treatments that require the transplantation of fully developed organs produced through stem cell therapy, prompting the production of millions of biologically precise coordinating cells. In order to incorporate such intricate processes into mainstream regenerative medicine, cooperation across disciplines and nations will be imperative.

Implemented as a fail-safe measure, one concept for enhancing the safety of stem cells involves incorporating a self-destruct mechanism in case of potential risks. The continued evolution and adaptability of stem cells have the potential to lower the expenses associated with treating individuals afflicted with presently incurable illnesses. In scenarios where organ failure is imminent, patients may opt for stem cell therapy instead of undergoing costly and intensive pharmaceutical interventions.

The benefits of a successful procedure would be immediate, enabling patients to avoid the need for prolonged pharmacological treatments and their associated side effects.

While the obstacles confronting the field of stem cell research may seem daunting, significant progress is being made on a daily basis. Stem cell therapy is currently being utilized to address a variety of medical conditions and ailments. The future implications of stem cells on the realm of medicine are poised to be substantial.

Organoids produced from stem cells sourced from adult animals

The term translational research, first introduced in the 1990s, actually has a history that dates back more than fifty years earlier. This concept promotes the utilization of animals as substitutes for studying human health and disease in the realms of biomedicine and pharmacology. [617]

Translational research has become a prevalent force in the field of biomedical research, although it is met with opposition stemming from concerns regarding the health and pain perception of experimental animals, as well as their overall well-being. Various regulatory bodies have been put in place to establish and enforce guidelines for the ethical treatment of animals in experiments. Despite these measures to enhance the welfare of research animals, there are still outstanding issues that must be tackled [618- **620**].

The Replacement principle advocates for the utilization of alternative non-animal models like in vitro or in silico methods, while the Reduction principle emphasizes the reduction of the quantity of animals utilized in experiments. Lastly, the Refinement principle aims to improve animal welfare and reduce suffering in research settings. In addition to ethical considerations, translational research also faces challenges in effectively translating results from animal models to humans, particularly in pharmacological efficacy and toxicity testing. [621, **622**].

Rodents are frequently utilized as a primary model in pharmacological research and have shown effectiveness in studying monogenetic diseases [623]. Nevertheless, doubts have been raised regarding the translational relevance of this model in the study of chronic multifactorial diseases. [623- **624**].

(1) The dietary model focuses solely on nutritional aspects while neglecting genetic and lifestyle influences.

(2) Although dietary modifications can improve the genetic model, it remains lacking in addressing other lifestyle factors.

(3) Conversely, the chemical model may factor in elements such as a high-fat diet, but it does not account for genetic variations or other lifestyle choices. [**626**]. As a result, rodents are not suitable for modeling complex multifactorial diseases that do not naturally manifest in their species. It is imperative for the scientific community to adopt innovative methods to study these diseases.

[**627**] The origins of the concept emerged during the early 1800s. It emphasizes the exchange of knowledge between human and veterinary medicine, with the overall goal of advancing biomedical research, enhancing clinical and paraclinical services, addressing biosafety concerns, and improving public health outcomes. A visual representation of the One Health Initiative is depicted in Figure 12A. This approach also aligns with the principles of the One Medicine approach.[627, 628]

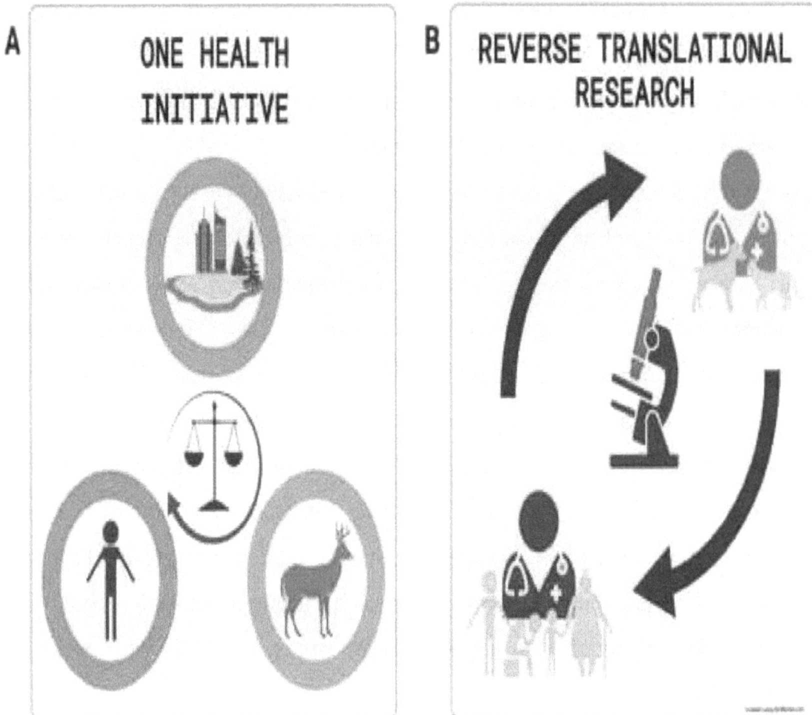

Figure 12 illustrates the One Health Initiative and Reverse Translational Research. The One Health Initiative is a pioneering method that strives to find holistic solutions to health challenges affecting humans, animals, and the environment, while also enhancing communication among researchers in the biomedical field. This approach is designed to enhance the field of biomedical science and create innovative research tactics. In line with the One Health Initiative, Reverse Translational Research encourages collaboration and information exchange between human and animal healthcare professionals and researchers in clinical and paraclinical settings. This concept emphasizes the sharing of pertinent patient data for translational research purposes.

In instances where veterinary patients exhibit a condition also found in the human population, their experiences can contribute valuable data on diagnostics, treatments, and outcomes that may ultimately enhance outcomes for human patients.

Similarly, knowledge gleaned from diseases investigated more extensively in human medicine can be applied to augment understanding and practices within veterinary medicine. A visual representation of the One Medicine methodology and the implications of reverse translational research can be observed in Figure 12B.

Reverse translational research offers significant benefits over conventional translational models. Key advantages include the similarities in animal domestication between companion animal patients and their owners, as well as their often sedentary lifestyles. Additionally, pet nutrition has mirrored human food processing trends for many years.

The rising prevalence of obesity in humans and their companion animals illustrates the impact of shared environmental factors. Through the integration of reverse translational research and advanced in vitro models, more reliable research instruments can be created that are less reliant on donor samples. [**630- 634**].

Moreover, the relevance of personalized and regenerative medicine is increasing as we gain more understanding of individualized treatment options for both animal and human patients. Prior to in vivo treatment, various drug candidates and their effects on the patient can be assessed in vitro at different concentrations. Personalized organoids hold promise for accelerating advancements in medical treatment. In addition to personalized drug testing, the areas of transplants and tissue repair have garnered significant attention in the field of organoids.

The most prevalent cell culture models used in vitro

Primary Cell Lines

Primary cell cultures can be directly extracted from a patient and utilized in a personalized medicine context. Nevertheless, the utilization of primary epithelial cell lines in biomedical research is accompanied by certain drawbacks that restrict their applicability. These challenges encompass the challenge of isolating singular cell types and the constrained longevity of the culture. The constrained longevity of cell lines significantly inhibits their utility, prompting numerous researchers to opt for commercially validated and immortalized cell lines. [**635**].

Diverse immortalized cell lines that have the capacity to continuously proliferate and uphold stability in their genetic makeup

Traditional two-dimensional cell cultures offer advantages in the field of biomedical research due to their convenience and low maintenance costs. Moreover, there is a significant amount of well-documented knowledge and experimentation accessible for these immortalized cell lines,. However, these models do present limitations, such as alterations in cellular morphology following isolation, which can impede the complexity of these cell models. [**635, 636**].

Cell lines derived from cancerous sources are typically utilized for in vitro intestinal permeability assays during drug testing. Despite this, these cellular monolayers are unable to fully replicate the complex physiological attributes of actual organs.

The Caco-2 cell line, established from human colorectal adenocarcinoma cells in 1977, serves as the gold standard for assessing intestinal permeability. [637, **638**].

While conducting experiments with Caco-2 cells offers a certain amount of data on intestinal permeability, it is important to note that this method is not without its limitations. Caco-2 cells are a single type of cell that has been altered and therefore do not present the diverse range of cell types found in a healthy intestine, such as goblet cells and enteroendocrine cells. [**639**].

Moreover, the permeability of Caco-2 cells is reduced as a result of changes in tight junction function in comparison to the intestinal tissue. [**637**, 640-**643**]

Organoids created from stem cells

Organoids are intricate, three-dimensional constructs created from stem cells that faithfully reproduce the microanatomy and physiological characteristics of individual organs.

This innovative technology has diverse applications in areas such as developmental biology, pathophysiology, drug development, toxicology, infectious disease research, and regenerative medicine. [644- **646**] (**Figure 13**).

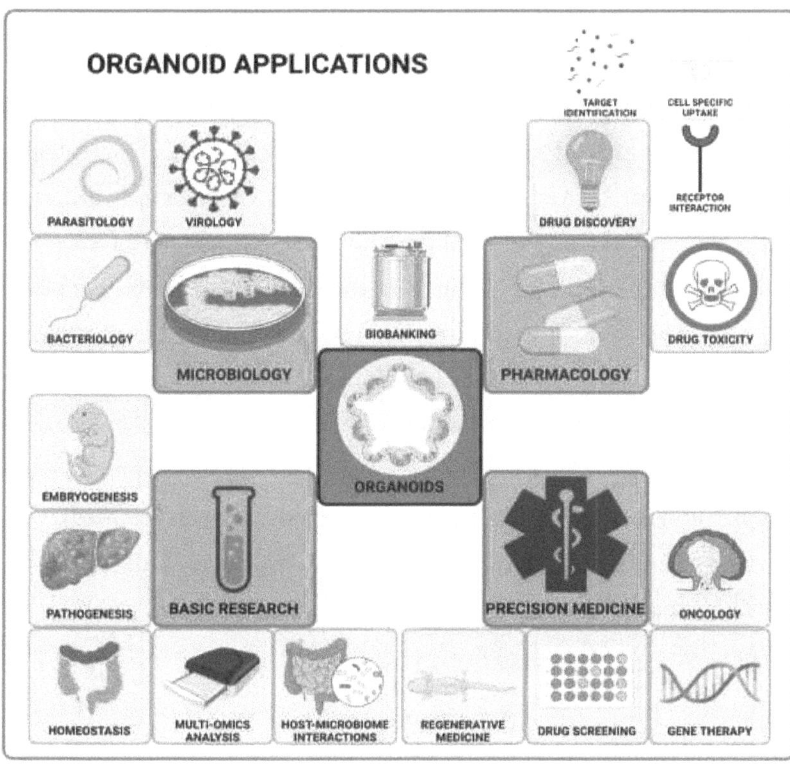

Figure 13 illustrates the various applications of organoids in the field of biomedical research. The dark orange frames highlight the main topics, the light orange frames indicate subfields, and the white frames outline specific applications. [**647**].

Pluripotent stem cell-derived organoids offer a valuable tool for exploring embryogenesis and tissue development. One key benefit of these organoids is that they contain cells representing all tissue layers found in living organisms.

On the other hand, organoids derived from adipose-derived stem cells are a more streamlined version of those derived from induced pluripotent stem cells. These organoids primarily consist of endodermal epithelial cell types but do not require the complicated process of reprogramming iPSCs. [648, **649**].

Adipose-derived stem cell (AdSC)-derived organoids have shown utility in modeling specific organs of endodermal origin. However, their application in replicating structures derived from ectodermal and mesodermal origins is restricted. In contrast, organoids derived from induced pluripotent stem cells (iPSCs) have vast potential for research in diverse fields such as cardiology, neurology, and bone disease. AdSC-derived organoids provide the advantage of continuous proliferation within a 3D culture system, offering the potential for long-term sample preservation through bioarchiving. [**646**]. Ultimately, these miniature organs can be formed without the need for embryonic cells and can be initiated from samples gathered through various biopsy methods, such as fine-needle, Tru-cut, or excisional samples, effectively meeting the requirements of the reverse translational approach.

Various extracellular membrane matrices can be used, with Matrigel, a basement membrane matrix in a soluble form, proving to be an advantageous environment for the growth and differentiation of organoids in a three-dimensional setting. These methodologies, sometimes with adjustments, have formed the core of current protocols for deriving organoids from adult stem cells.

The isolation techniques for different tissues have followed a similar approach, often involving the use of distinct markers for detecting stem cells (for example, EpCAM for the liver). Moreover, Zdyrski et al. documented the isolation of diverse tissues from dogs using the same methodologies, which contributed to the standardization of these procedures. [645- **652**].

Organoid cultures have been successfully developed from a range of species, with a particular emphasis on mammalian organoids. This article will concentrate on organoids sourced from Adipose-derived Stem Cells (AdSC) due to the significant amount of research in this field. The discussion will include human and rodent organoids to provide context for the progression of organoid research. Furthermore, the introduction will primarily examine the uses of organoids derived from healthy animals [653, 654] Figure 14 provides an overview of the chronological progression of human and animal organoid formation.

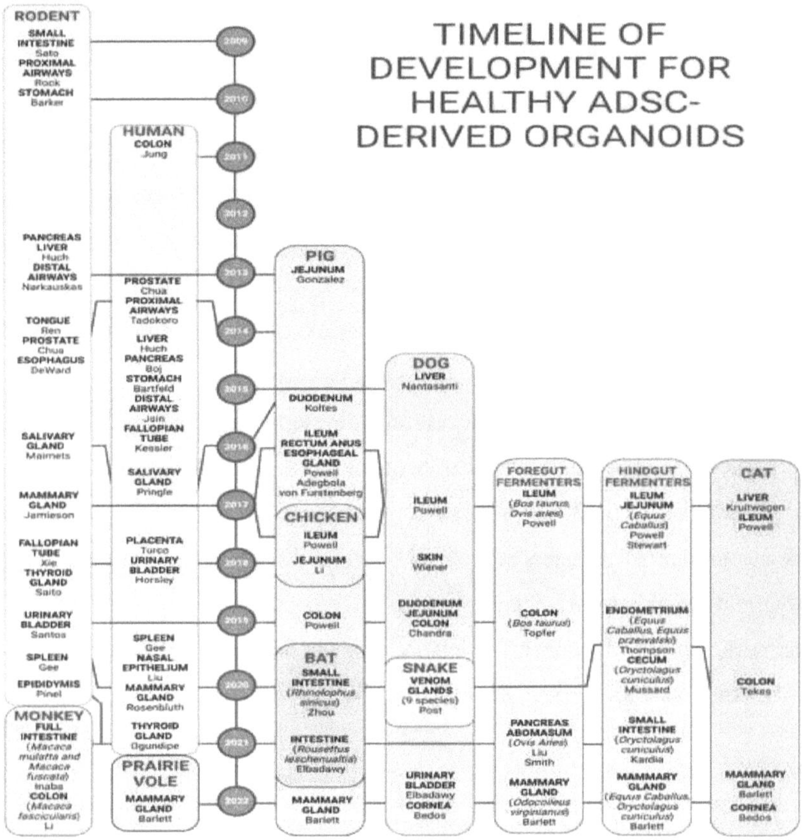

Figure 14 illustrates the chronological progression of the development of organoids derived from AdSC. The timeline encompasses the initial documentation of organoid formation in various species, spanning from humans and rodents to a diverse array of animals, both common and exotic, within the field of veterinary medicine. Reproducibility and Data Deposition

The field of organoid (stem cell) research is continuously evolving within the realm of biomedical research. The advancement of this field faces challenges due to the absence of standardized practices, particularly within the context of veterinary medicine. Despite ongoing initiatives to create uniform In the realm of veterinary organoid cultures, the significance of maintaining uniform data and methodologies is readily apparent. Precise delineation of organoid markers, species and individual differences, as well as the developmental phase of the organoids is essential in laying the groundwork for this field. [**655**].

A related issue in terms of replicability pertains to the hydrogels utilized in stem cell culturing, which frequently contain unspecified components derived from animals and exhibit inconsistencies between different production batches. [**656**].

Organoids derived from human cells

The extraction and nurturing of human colon-derived organoids, commonly referred to as colonoids, from adult stem cells is a significant achievement in scientific research. [686-**700**].

Although human-derived organoids offer a promising opportunity to replicate human in vivo settings with precision, there exist multiple complications associated with this technology. The availability of donors is restricted, and the ethical implications of obtaining healthy tissue raise concerns. Ethical dilemmas extend beyond the realm of organoid technology to encompass its integration with other methodologies, including the development of chimeras, gene editing of organoids, trials involving organoid transplantation, and the commercialization of human-derived technology. The notable constraints in conducting in vivo experiments on donors further impede progress in pathophysiological and pharmaceutical research.[701]

Murine Organoids

Rodents are commonly used as experimental models in biomedical research, with mice being the most prevalent species utilized and a diverse array of genetically modified strains readily available.

Additionally, their widespread use, cost-effective maintenance, and high reproductive rate make them one of the most cost-efficient animal models for research studies. The in-depth understanding of donor rodent physiology and the ability to compare results with past in vivo experiments make murine organoids a preferred choice for translational research. [702- **714**].

The common utilization of mice as a research model is due to their cost-effectiveness and the wide range of genetic variations accessible. Nonetheless, there are disadvantages to utilizing mice, including their shorter lifespans which can impede the examination of chronic illnesses and non-naturally transpiring conditions. These constraints have the potential to confine the relevance of conclusions drawn from mouse studies to different species. Despite progress in murine organoids offering hope for translational research, the possibilities for reverse translational applications in mice are restricted. [**624**].

Additional organoids derived from animal sources

Over the past decade, there have been a multitude of species, both exotic and traditional veterinary animals, that have been effectively employed for organoid culture growth through adaptations of protocols originally designed for human and murine cells. These cell lines, once successfully established, have often served as foundational evidence for the potential application of animal-derived organoids in various biomedical fields. [**639, 715**].

In 2017, Powell and colleagues conducted a study to explore the feasibility of establishing organoids from various species within the animal kingdom. The research revealed significant conservation in protein sequences of Key growth factors like Wnt3a, R-spondin, and Noggin have been identified in various species, including humans, rodents, and a diverse array of animals such as dogs, cats, cows, horses, pigs, goats, sheep, and chickens. This genetic likeness allows for the promotion of organoid development in non-murine species utilizing growth factors from mice and humans. [672]

The development of organoids from unconventional animal species has the potential to enhance the understanding of unique physiologies, environments, and disease processes within the original species. While these cell lines may not always be applicable in reverse translational research, they align with the objectives of the One Health Initiative.[680]

Nevertheless, there is a widespread belief that organoids originating from extensively researched veterinary species exhibit the most promise for application in reverse translational research. A comprehensive understanding of medical data and research discoveries pertaining to these species is essential.

Furthermore, the impact of domestication, characterized by stringent phenotypic selection and ongoing interaction with humans, holds great significance. The domestication process fundamentally alters the environment and dietary patterns of animals to mirror those of humans. [716, **717**].

In 2021, Beaumont and his team released an in-depth analysis discussing the progress made in creating organoid models derived from pigs, ruminants, horses, and chickens. The study delves into a range of research endeavors, detailing the methodologies involved in the isolation and cultivation of these organoids. [**718**].

Companion animals, or pet animals, belonging to the veterinary species, often reside within the same household environment as their owners. Their dietary needs are often adjusted to mirror human food consumption, and they may adopt similar lifestyle habits such as a sedentary routine. One area of significant promise in reverse translational research lies in the development of canine organoids.

The Food and Drug Administration recognizes the value of clinical trials involving dogs, deeming their results to be of higher quality than those obtained from rodent studies, especially within the realm of translational research. The field of canine medicine is at the forefront of veterinary research, producing vast amounts of data that have the potential to be applied to human medicine. With all these factors considered, canines emerge as an ideal target for further exploration in reverse translational research. [**630, 639, 719**].

In the last ten years, there has been significant progress in the development of canine organoid technology. Published methodologies for creating intestinal and hepatic organoids have become more refined, and new organoid varieties have been identified. This article examines the potential uses of various organoid culture systems, emphasizing the research possibilities offered by organoids derived from animals. [**639,682**].

Main Research Applications

Intestinal organoids serve as a valuable tool for investigating intestinal functionality across a range of species. In 2021, Inaba et al. achieved success in generating monkey intestinal organoids from various regions of the gastrointestinal tract, including the duodenum, jejunum, ileum, cecum, and colon. By utilizing a rhesus monkey (Macaca mulatta) and a Japanese macaque (Macaca fuscata), the researchers were able to sustain the growth of these organoids for a duration of six months. The methodology employed in this study adhered to the guidelines for establishing murine intestinal organoids as proposed by Mahe et al. in 2013. [720].

In 2021, Li and colleagues conducted a research study documenting the development of colonic organoids from two cynomolgus monkeys, also referred to as crab-eating monkeys (Macaca fascicularis). The scientists followed the method for isolating human colonic stem cells outlined by Jung and others in 2011 to initiate the cultivation process. In order to achieve the ultimate differentiation of the cultured cells, they decreased the levels of CHIR-99021 (a GSK-3 inhibitor) and ceased the presence of prostaglandin E2 (PGE2) to reduce Wnt signaling. [660]

Extended exposure of organoids to these specified conditions was observed to result in cell death. Li et al. conducted a week-long maintenance of the organoids in differentiation media before conducting an analysis of the culture. Their research findings demonstrated the successful differentiation of enterocytes and goblet cells in the medium, although the promotion of differentiation in enteroendocrine cells was not as successful.

Further investigation is necessary to examine the developmental stage and functional attributes of these organoids. Just like in humans, the elimination of Wnt3a was crucial for cell differentiation and maturation; however, it caused the macaque intestinal organoid culture to collapse.

Moreover, the media was modified by removing SB202190 (a P38 MAPK inhibitor) and nicotinamide to enhance differentiation. Inaba et al. studied the differentiation of intestinal taste-like chemosensory cells, such as enteroendocrine and tuft cells, in culture by incorporating interleukin 4 (IL-4) and the Notch inhibitor dibenzazepine (DBZ). [660]

The researchers conducted an analysis of organoid expression and chemoreception responses, leading to the conclusion that taste-like chemosensory cells derived from monkeys exhibit functional similarities to those found in humans rather than rodents.

In a recent study conducted by Inaba and colleagues (2021), notable progress was achieved in the field of monkey intestinal culture methods. [721- **725**].

In 2020, Acharya and colleagues developed a novel technique for growing galline small intestinal organoids, with a specific focus on the duodenum and jejunum. Their method involved omitting the use of extracellular matrix for structural support, reducing the need for growth factors during the establishment of organoid culture, and nurturing the organoids in an apical-out arrangement. The researchers extracted and processed mucosa from fresh tissue through extrusion, trituration, and centrifugation. The resultant pellet was then suspended in a solution comprising fetal bovine serum (FBS), insulin transferrin selenite (ITS), polyamine (likely derived from intestinal bacteria in vivo), and bovine pituitary extract, and allowed to grow overnight. [674]

The treatment initiated a repair mechanism in the damaged portions of the villi, leading to the formation of organoids. The cultivated enteroids were then processed and utilized for further experiments. The researchers observed a beneficial impact on the organoid culture with the addition of growth factors such as EGF and IGF-1. Although not classified as a prolonged organoid culture, the techniques utilized in this study could potentially be used to develop efficient and affordable culture systems independent of extracellular matrix components in the future.

The organoids were examined using transmission electron microscopy (TEM), which clearly showed microvilli present on the apical surface. Furthermore, reverse transcription polymerase chain reaction (RT-PCR) was employed to identify stem cell marker genes like OlfM4, Znrf3, Hopx, and LGR5. To visually assess the viability of the organoids, neutral red staining was utilized, and an EdU assay was conducted to confirm their ability to proliferate.

In 2019, Töpfer and colleagues introduced bovine colon-derived organoids using a protocol established by Sato for human intestinal organoids in 2011. The colonoids displayed impressive proliferative capabilities, maintaining viability through over 30 passages. Differentiation of these organoids was achieved by incorporating DAPT for 24 hours, resulting in decreased LGR5 expression and increased expression of mucin2, chromogranin A, and CA1 markers, indicating the presence of goblet cells, enteroendocrine cells, and enterocytes.

In a novel experiment, researchers utilized bovine organoids for an in situ cryopreservation study. The organoids were frozen on a plate without harvesting, utilizing cryopreservation media, and stored at -150 °C for 24 hours. Upon thawing, the culture demonstrated growth comparable to traditionally preserved unfrozen controls. Subsequent cytotoxicity assays with staurosporine as a stimulant showed no significant difference in average toxicity between cryopreserved samples and controls. Bioprinting applications were also explored, with bovine organoids successfully forming 2D monolayers on dual-chamber permeable supports. Further investigation of these organoid models is recommended for future research endeavors. [665,645, 666, 668, 725]

In 2020, Mussard et al. were the first to pioneer the development of rabbit cecal organoids. Their study involved a thorough examination of different growth media options, incorporating various pharmacological inhibitors such as a GSK-3 inhibitor for activating the Wnt pathway and LDN193189, a bone morphogenic pathway inhibitor, in the absence of WRN. [**667**].

The results suggest that the growth of rabbit cecum organoids is not solely dependent on the activation of the Wnt pathway, unlike human organoids which require a GSK-3 inhibitor for activation. In the specific media used, there was an observed increase in the proliferation of the organoids. [726,**727**].

Two distinct types of organoids were identified in the culture: hollow/ductal spheroids, which were characterized by the presence of cytokeratin 7, and solid squamous spheroids, which were distinguished by abundant P63. Both varieties of spheroids exhibited a high rate of proliferation and were dependent on epidermal growth factor. Adegbola et al. successfully generated porcine anorectal organoids in 2017 to serve as a model for perianal fistulas in Crohn's disease.

While the rectal organoids showed a phenotype similar to those derived from the small intestine, organoids from the anal and anorectal transition zones displayed a monolayer phenotype. [669]

In 2019, Chandra and colleagues introduced the innovative concept of canine intestinal organoid culture. They modified the methodology initially developed by Saxena and his team in 2015 for human intestinal organoids to create organoids that exhibit the characteristics of different segments of the canine intestine, such as the duodenum, jejunum, ileum, and colon. Canine enteroid and colonoid lines were successfully established from a group of twenty-eight healthy canines and twelve animals with various health conditions, including inflammatory bowel disease (IBD), gastrointestinal stromal tumor (GIST), colorectal adenocarcinoma, and animal models of lysosomal storage disease (MPS type 1). [**728, 729**].

In their study, the authors contrasted the qPCR markers NEUROG3 and chromogranin A to illustrate a congruent differentiation pattern in organoids cultured in refined versus expansion media. The use of refined medium led to a notable fourfold rise in organoid count when compared to expansion medium. Although the refined media formulation displayed encouraging outcomes, the authors emphasized the need for additional experimentation with a larger sample size to verify and enhance their findings. [**731**, **732**].

Furthermore, the integrity of the intestinal barrier was confirmed using immunofluorescence staining to detect zonula occludens 1 and E-cadherin, as well as evaluating monolayer transepithelial electrical resistance (TEER). The crucial efflux pump, P-gp, was identified on the apical surface of the monolayer and its presence was verified through functional experiments. Ambrosini et al. demonstrated the successful establishment and characterization of canine intestinal cultures in a permeable dual-chamber system.

The subsequent demonstration of the progress in organoid technology for evaluating drug permeability and toxicity involves its integration into a microfluidic system. Microfluidic channels are introduced within organoids, and the flow of media within these channels mimics the circulation of blood in the body. By exposing the organoids to the physiological shear stress experienced in the body, this method provides an additional advantage. Additionally, the inclusion of coculture chambers enables the mimicry of interactions between organoid cultures and other organs or the immune system. The potential next step for this technology involves investigating hepatocyte differentiation within a microfluidic chip. [733]

Modeling Host-Pathogen Interactions

Animal-derived organoids have shown promise in the field of host-pathogen interactions research. Although intestinal organoids have been commonly utilized for this purpose, researchers have proposed utilizing lung or abomasum-derived organoids as well.

[734]

In 2017, Powell and Behnke successfully isolated ileal porcine organoids along with duodenal and jejunal counterparts to serve as a host-pathogen model.

These organoids were sustained using L-WRN medium and were able to survive in culture for 174 days.

In 2019, Li et al. introduced a groundbreaking approach to studying porcine epidemic diarrhea virus (PEDV) infection using porcine colonoids. These researchers infected ileal and colonic organoids from a single donor with PEDV, observing that the ileal organoids were susceptible to infection without restrictions, whereas the colonoids only showed limited susceptibility. Additionally, the ileal enteroids contained a notably higher amount of viral genome copies compared to the colonoids.

A previous study on infected piglets had highlighted differences in junction alterations between the small intestine and the colon, indicating that porcine intestinal organoids retain the unique characteristics of their specific intestinal segment, as emphasized by Li et al.[735]

Powell and colleagues, in 2017, detailed the initial galline cecal organoids developed using a 50% concentration of L-WRN-conditioned media. The establishment of these organoid lines involved six individuals, achieving a success rate of 66%, with the highest passage number reaching 35, equivalent to approximately 125 days of cultivation. These organoids exhibited minimal vimentin expression, indicative of their ability to function independently of mesenchymal cells within the coculture setting, and displayed notably elevated levels of LGR5, a marker for stem cells and progenitors, compared to that observed in the corresponding tissue samples.

The first bovine ileal organoids were characterized in 2017, originating from five different donors. Sustained growth and expansion of the organoids were facilitated through the use of L-WRN medium, allowing for passage up to 45 times (approximately 165 days). The enteroids showcased comparable levels of LGR5, a marker for stem cells, to those present in native tissue. Conversely, conventional bovine cell cultures utilized in intestinal research, such as the Madin-Darby bovine kidney cell line, lacked detectable expression of LGR5. Notably, MDBK cells were selected for their capacity to emulate the tight junction and barrier properties of the intestinal monolayer. Powell and colleagues, in 2017, detailed the initial galline cecal organoids developed using a 50% concentration of L-WRN-conditioned media. The establishment of these organoid lines involved six individuals, achieving a success rate of 66%, with the highest passage number reaching 35, equivalent to approximately 125 days of cultivation. These organoids exhibited minimal vimentin expression, indicative of their ability to function independently of mesenchymal cells within the coculture setting, and displayed notably elevated levels of LGR5, a marker for stem cells and progenitors, compared to that observed in the corresponding tissue samples.

The first bovine ileal organoids were characterized in 2017, originating from five different donors. Sustained growth and expansion of the organoids were facilitated through the use of L-WRN medium, allowing for passage up to 45 times (approximately 165 days). The enteroids showcased comparable levels of LGR5, a marker for stem cells, to those present in native tissue. Conversely, conventional bovine cell cultures utilized in intestinal research, such as the Madin-Darby bovine kidney cell line, lacked detectable expression of LGR5. Notably, MDBK cells were selected for their capacity to emulate the tight junction and barrier properties of the intestinal monolayer. [672]

In 2019, Derricott et al. developed bovine jejunal enteroids as a tool for examining host-pathogen interactions and disease responses. [**675, 672**].

The cultures were established using samples from four donors and were able to reach 66 passages, equivalent to 239 days of growth. In the organoids, there was a higher expression of LGR5 RNA compared to the control tissue, and the low presence of vimentin (a mesenchymal marker) indicated that mesenchymal cells may not be essential for the expansion of the organoids. This observation is consistent with findings in other veterinary species. [**718, 737**].

The researchers investigated the invasive capabilities of the full parasite Teladorsagia circumcincta in organoid cultures. Observations revealed that within a day of introducing the parasite, it was able to penetrate the Matrigel and successfully invade the organoids.

After fourteen days in culture, motile worms could still be found within the culture.

The study findings led the authors to conclude that parasitic pathogens have the capacity to infiltrate organoids, suggesting potential applications for modeling host-pathogen interactions. Further examination in this area is recommended to deepen our understanding. [737]

In 2020, Tekes et al. performed a research study regarding the most effective methods for sustaining feline ileal and colonic organoids in extended cultures. The objective of this study was to examine feline coronaviruses, specifically feline enteric coronavirus (FECV) and the fatal feline infectious peritonitis virus (FIPV). [**678**].

The cultivated organoid culture was evaluated using quantitative polymerase chain reaction (qPCR), which indicated the presence of all cellular components found in the intestine. Interestingly, the colonic tissue showed no expression of Lyz, a known marker for Paneth cells. Several methodologies for passaging feline intestinal cultures were investigated, including trypsinization, mechanical disruption, and gentle cell dissociation reagents. It was concluded that mechanical disruption is the most efficient technique for producing organoids with the greatest diameter.

An alternative study was carried out to assess the development of organoids in traditional human and mouse media. Results indicated that cells from the ileum and colon flourished more effectively in human media. Nonetheless, neither cell cultures from these organs were able to sustain FIPV growth, while ileal organoids were found to be unsupportive of FECV growth. On the other hand, feline colonic organoids were able to support FECV infection, suggesting their potential utility in further research on feline coronaviral infections. .

Liver Organoids

The importance of organoids in modeling disease lies in the ability to create organoids specific to individual patients using biopsies. Furthermore, the ability to correct potential disease-causing mutations allows for investigation of cause and effect. The artificial environment in which organoids are grown, with high levels of growth factors, oxygen, and nutrients, as well as the absence of interaction with other cell types, necessitates careful consideration when comparing results obtained in vitro with those seen in vivo.

In 2015, Nantasanti et al. first developed hepatic-derived organoids from canines for investigative purposes. These organoids proved to be a valuable tool for studying gene therapy related to Wilson's disease, a condition not commonly seen in dogs. Through inducing a similar pathophysiology in dogs deficient in COMMD1, researchers were able to replicate harmful copper accumulation in the liver. The study underscored the significant presence of stem cell characteristics in the organoids, underscoring the necessity of refining hepatocyte differentiation techniques. Additionally, the research showcased successful correction of the genetic anomaly linked to COMMD1 deficiency and subsequent liver copper accumulation through lentiviral transduction of the entire COMMD1 gene sequence. [**682**]

These hepatic stem cells, which were genetically corrected to match each individual dog, were transplanted into recipient dogs with a deficiency in COMMD1 through the portal vein. The animals were able to survive for a minimum of two years; however, upon integration into the liver, there was a lack of notable cell proliferation and no improvement in copper accumulation and biliary copper excretion. Organoids were developed using liver samples from both healthy dogs and those with congenital portosystemic shunts (CPSS). When these organoids were cultured in a medium containing high levels of free fatty acids, they demonstrated similar steatosis characteristics commonly observed in CPSS livers. [738, **739**].

Disease modeling can be exemplified by the examination of canine liver organoids obtained from both healthy dogs and those with a deficiency in COMMD1, as well as organoids from COMMD1-deficient dogs that have undergone repair, which have been shown to display reduced FXR transcriptional activity. This finding aligns with observations made in copper-loaded human livers.

In a recent study conducted in 2022, further investigation into canine hepatic organoids was discussed, focusing on the standardization of canine hepatic and intestinal cultures. The current lack of standardized protocols for handling procedures in adult-derived canine organoid technology poses a challenge for comparing research both within and between laboratories, mainly due to its recent introduction. The protocols for canine organoids are primarily based on the methodologies outlined in studies by Saxena et al. (2015) involving human intestinal organoids infected with rotavirus, and a subsequent protocol developed by Zou et al. in 2019. [740,**741**]

The research team outlined three distinct procedures for the management of organoid cultures, which include the establishment, maintenance, and harvesting of the organoids. The initial step, referred to as the Canine Organoid Isolation Protocol, involves the process of obtaining samples and embedding tissue suspensions. The Canine Organoid Maintenance protocol details the necessary steps to ensure the proper growth and maintenance of the organoid culture, such as cleaning and passaging of the organoids. Lastly, the Canine Organoid Harvesting and Biobanking Protocol provides guidance on preparing organoid cultures for various applications, including fixation, archival in liquid nitrogen, and preservation of RNA samples.

In 2017, Kruitwagen et al. created and characterized feline hepatic organoids for the purpose of studying hepatic steatosis. The researchers utilized five feline hepatic biopsies, which were obtained from fresh, frozen, and fine-needle aspirates. The organoid culture reached a passage number of 25, demonstrating durability and stability. [**742**].

Based on a experimental study on free fatty acid accumulation, two potential drug candidates were discovered, mirroring the approach taken by Kruitwagen et al. in 2017. These drugs were found to reduce the buildup of triacylglycerol in both differentiated (hepatocyte-like) and undifferentiated (cholangiocyte) hepatic organoids. As a result, the researchers suggest that differentiation may not necessarily be a crucial initial stage, and screening of undifferentiated organoids could prove beneficial in drug discovery efforts.

Renal Organoids

The MDCK cell line, also referred to as the Madine-Darby canine kidney cell line, is widely recognized as one of the most utilized canine cell lines in scientific research. Unlike the extensive studies conducted on this renowned cell line, there is a scarcity of information available on canine kidney organoids, with only a single publication addressing this subject.

The authors of this publication underscore the significance of organoids in biomedical research pertaining to end-stage renal disease, as well as stressing the necessity for ideal culture conditions, such as the incorporation of N-acetylcysteine, ascorbic acid 2-phosphate, nicotinamide, and fetal bovine serum (FBS). Additionally, Chen et al. conducted a comparison study between their organoid culture and the conventional MDCK 2D culture that was originally introduced in 1958. [**743**].

After being cultured in Matrigel, multipotent canine kidney cells with characteristics similar to mesenchymal stem cells (MSCs) displayed the formation of tubule-like structures. The expression of CD24 and CD133 in these cells aligns with the known markers for renal adipose-derived stem cells (ASCs), but their MSC-like features suggest a closer resemblance to MSCs rather than adult kidney stem cells. Renal ASCs induced with Wnt-stimulating media were found to maintain CD24 and CD133 expression, yet lacked the ability to differentiate into adipogenic, chondrogenic, or osteoblastic lineages. [**661**].

Pancreatic Organoids

The investigation of pancreatic organoids has the potential to provide valuable insights into the functionality and abnormalities of this essential organ. A notable research study carried out by Liu et al. in the year 2021 delved into the effects of copper supplementation on the ovine pancreas. The researchers discovered that copper supplementation played a critical role in the development of pancreatic organoids, a phenomenon previously observed in a different in vivo study where copper deficiency led to neurological issues in newborns and non-specific symptoms in adults. By following a protocol for isolating primary pancreatic cells from rodents developed by Agbunag et al. in 2006, the authors extracted pancreatic ducts from a fetal sheep and conducted their experiments. [744, **745**].

The pancreatic organoids displayed characteristics reminiscent of pancreatic epithelial progenitors, and were also found to express additional stem cell markers such as LGR5 and EPCAM. The lack of expression of endocrine cell markers like insulin, glucagon, and amylase resulted in the designation of these organoids as "sheep pancreatic duct organoids", due to their high level of cytokeratin 19, a marker for ductal cells. Incorporating RSPO1 and EGF into the organoid culture medium was determined to be essential, as the presence of more cyst-like organoids was observed in the supplemented medium compared to the control. This observation was confirmed through both the EdU proliferation assay and the CCK8 viability assay. Furthermore, the researchers conducted a forskolin-induced swelling assay to showcase CFTR activity, and a chloride movement assay to verify the functional characteristics of the organoids.

The introduction of the copper chelator tetrathiomolybdate into the medium during an experiment led to the inhibition of organoid formation and growth, a finding that was validated by a CCK8 assay. Adequate growth of the organoids was observed with the appropriate supplementation of copper at a concentration of 10 μM. Conversely, an excess of copper supplementation at 100 μM had a significant negative impact on organoid growth. These results were supported by both EdU and CCK8 assays. Additionally, the researchers explored the role of the MEK-ERK pathway in mediating the effects of copper on organoids and further investigated copper interactions using a knockdown organoid model.

SARS-COVID-2

The emergence of the SARS-COVID-2 pandemic prompted a thorough examination of coronaviral infections, leading to the development of two model organoid lines that were specifically created to aid in the study of the disease. In 2020, Zhou et al. produced bat enteroids utilizing a protocol initially established for deriving human intestinal organoids in 2011 by Sato et al.

The primary focus of the researchers was to investigate the infection caused by SARS-COVID-2 in an intestinal bat model. This interest stemmed from early research suggesting a potential link between the pandemic and a host species known as the horseshoe bat (Rhinolophus sinicus). [**746**].

Zhou and colleagues demonstrated that bat enteroids are vulnerable to COVID-19 infection, and the virus is able to reproduce within these organoids. This groundbreaking finding offers proof of SARS-CoV-2's capability to invade bat intestinal cells. The researchers acknowledged their inability to sustain long-term organoid expansion as per Sato's established protocol, indicating the necessity for further refinement of the methodology. Additionally, Zhou et al. highlighted the presence of several potentially zoonotic viruses in the bat intestine, emphasizing the utility of bat organoids for investigating such pathogens.

In a recent study published in 2021, Elbadawy and team detailed the creation of intestine-derived organoids from Leschenault's rousette fruit bat (Rousettus leschenaultia). [**681**].

The researchers successfully determined the optimal culture conditions for the long-term expansion of the culture. They conducted an experiment that demonstrated the critical role of Wnt, R-Spondin, Noggin (collectively known as WRN), transforming growth factor alpha (TGF-α), and epidermal growth factor (EGF) in sustaining the growth and proliferation of organoids. While the intestinal organoids showed resilience against SARS-CoV-2, they exhibited sensitivity to Pteropine orthoreovirus (PRV) inoculation. Elbadawy and colleagues proposed the potential use of bat intestinal organoids for investigating various rousette bat-related viruses, including Ebola or Marburg virus.

Precision/Personalized Medicine

Elbadawy and colleagues conducted a study to explore the application of organoid technology in the context of precision medicine for individuals with bladder cancer. Their findings indicate that this research has potential implications for treating bladder cancer in canines. [**747**].

Other Applications

Reproductive Physiology and Pathology

Animal-derived organoids have been developed for the purpose. Successfully created equine uterine organoids from biopsies taken from a total of 14 adult domestic and Przewalski's mares. These organoids were found to produce mucin, as indicated by PAS staining, and were also tested for their response to hormonal stimuli.

The development of organoids derived from a Przewalski's horse marked a significant milestone as it represented the first instance of organoids created from an endangered species. This achievement underscores the potential for studying biological processes in endangered species without the need to harm or sacrifice the animals. Furthermore, research has shown that prolactin has the ability to stimulate the synthesis of beta-casein in equine mammary organoids, shedding light on their functional properties. Although horses are not conventionally used for milk production, they serve as a valuable animal model for studying lactation mechanisms and allowing for comparisons across species. [659]

Estradiol-17β was discovered to have a suppressive effect on ESR1 gene expression in both frozen and fresh tissue-derived organoids. Conversely, the expression of PGR gene exhibited an increase in organoids derived from fresh tissue. Surprisingly, the response of the organoids to hormonal fluctuations did not align with expectations and did not replicate the reactions observed in living organisms. The researchers proposed that there may be a missing element in the feedback loop for gene regulation, or that the diffusion of hormones through the extracellular matrix could be compromised. In addition, Thompson and his colleagues conducted a study on cryopreservation, evaluating the growth rate, cellular viability, and other attributes of organoids derived from equine endometrium. [**748**].

Thompson and colleagues expanded their study on equine organoids by incorporating a protocol for equine oviductal organoids. The culture was maintained for a period of 42 days and underwent three passages. Additional exploration of this model is deemed necessary. The authors suggest leveraging organoid technology to propel research in artificial reproductive techniques.

In feline endometrial organoids, there was evidence of polarization and laminin expression in the basement membrane. This organoid system was initially developed to evaluate the toxicity of plastics or explore the potential for new antibiotics, thus details on cellular differentiation were not provided. [749, **750**].

Skin Diseases

The development of scar tissue on the skin due to injury can have social implications and negatively impact the quality of life. As a result, there has been a push for research in skin organoids, including the creation of canine skin organoids. Tissue samples were collected from twelve donors between the ages of 1-2 years who had been euthanized for reasons unrelated to this study. Utilizing microdissection techniques outlined in previous literature, the authors extracted hair follicles and the interfollicular epidermis. Each sample was then processed individually for every dog. The follicles and epidermis underwent digestion with collagenase 1A and II, hyaluronidase, and followed by overnight trypsinization to create a suspension of single-cell keratinocytes. After straining, the cells were cultivated in Matrigel for further studies. [751]

Immunohistochemistry and gene expression profiling validated the proliferative nature of Estradiol-17β was discovered to have a suppressive effect on

ESR1 gene expression in both frozen and fresh tissue-derived organoids. Conversely, the expression of PGR gene exhibited an increase in organoids derived from fresh tissue. Surprisingly, the response of the organoids to hormonal fluctuations did not align with expectations and did not replicate the reactions observed in living organisms. The researchers proposed that there may be a missing element in the feedback loop for gene regulation, or that the diffusion of hormones through the extracellular matrix could be compromised. In addition, Thompson and his colleagues conducted a study on cryopreservation, evaluating the growth rate, cellular viability, and other attributes of organoids derived from equine endometrium.

The majority of organoid cultures obtained from follicles or the epidermis exhibited a limited expansion capacity, typically lasting between six to fifteen passages, although one exception was noted where an organoid line persisted for up to 50 passages without reliance on A-83-01, a TGF-β inhibitor. [**752**].

The most unexpected discovery was that IFE-derived organoids grown in expansion medium (EM) mirrored the layered skin architecture.

Ophthalmology

Advancements in stem cell technology have recently been observed in the realm of veterinary ophthalmology. In a groundbreaking study by Bedos et al. in 2022, corneal organoids were successfully developed from canine and feline tissue, marking a significant milestone in the field [685]. The presence of crucial corneal epithelial and stromal cell markers was confirmed in the organoids through the utilization of the RNA in situ hybridization technique. This groundbreaking achievement marked the first instance of isolating corneal organoids from adult stem cells in any species. Although the experiment yielded promising results in the formation of organoid structures, further research is necessary to enhance the growth conditions of the culture.

Antivenom Production

The production of antivenom relies on the availability of snake venom obtained through a process known as "venom milking". This procedure involves a skilled herpetologist inducing a venomous snake to bite onto a plastic membrane over a collection jar in order to prompt the expulsion of venom from its fangs for collection. The techniques for extracting venom and housing snakes have seen gradual enhancements over the course of the last hundred years. Provide a comprehensive analysis in their review on the evolution of venomous snake housing at the Brazilian Butantan Institute since 1908. [**753**].

The toxin extracted during the collection process is used to immunize laboratory animals, mainly horses. Following this, blood or plasma is gathered, and the effective immunoglobulin elements are refined. The production of antivenom is a painstaking and expensive undertaking, with varying levels of output leading to insecurity in the availability of antivenom.

The mortality rate linked to snake bites is estimated to be around 125,000 fatalities annually, emphasizing the urgent need for innovative solutions in antivenom treatment. [754-**756**].

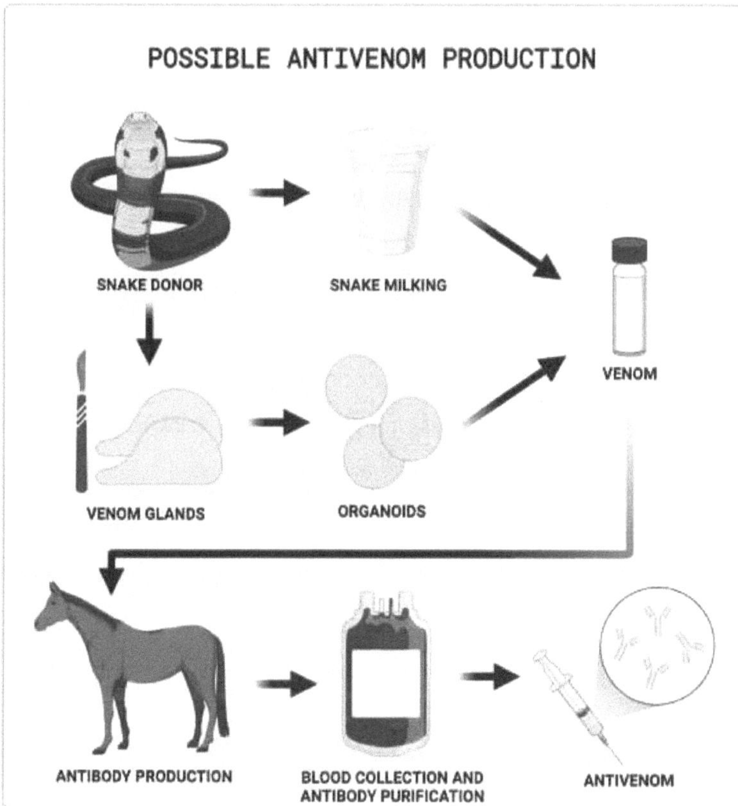

Figure 15. Potential method for producing antivenom involves utilizing snake venom gland organoids as a substitute for the arduous process of snake milking. By introducing venom into an animal, the immunized animal can generate antibodies. Subsequently, the animal's blood would be harvested, and the antibodies could be isolated and refined to create the ultimate product—antivenom.

In 2020, Post et al. conducted a study outlining the creation of organoids extracted from the venom glands of nine different snake species. These newly developed organoids were found to produce venom peptides that accurately reflected the composition and biological properties of the corresponding crude venom. The utilization of snake-derived organoids could potentially revolutionize the process of venom extraction for the production of antivenom, ultimately replacing the hazardous practice of venom milking.

This groundbreaking research has the additional distinction of establishing the first organoids belonging to the Reptilia class. Post et al. recognized the critical role of Wnt signaling in the growth of reptile organoids, a finding that parallels the importance of this signaling pathway in organoids derived from mammalian species. The successful establishment of organoid lines was facilitated by the addition of the Wnt pathway agonist R-spondin to the culture media. The authors propose that the growth conditions established for organoids in general could potentially be applied to all vertebrate species. [**654**].

Application of mesenchymal stem cells for the rehabilitation of tendons in the fields of veterinary and human medicine

Energy-storing tendons play a crucial role in facilitating efficient motion by utilizing stretch and recoil mechanisms, but they are also subjected to intense loading situations that result in high levels of stress and strain during physical activities. Consequently, these tendons are vulnerable to injuries caused by excessive strain. Among all the energy-storing tendons found in the human body, the Achilles tendon, also known as the calcaneal tendon, is both essential for energy transfer and highly susceptible to damage. This particular tendon is often associated with the popular expression "Achilles' heel," which signifies a person's vulnerable point. [758, 759]

The Achilles tendon has the function of connecting the plantaris, gastrocnemius, and soleus muscles to the calcaneus, is enveloped by a bursa on both sides, and allows for the flexion of the foot. [758, 759]

The canine common calcaneal tendon (CCT) bears striking resemblance in both composition and function to the human Achilles tendon, making it a valuable model for studying Achilles tendon injuries in humans. Comprised of the gastrocnemius tendon, superficial digital flexor tendon (SDFT), and common tendons of the biceps femoris, gracilis, and semitendinosis muscles, the CCT attaches to the calcaneus bone, encased by a bursa, and plays a crucial role in extending the tarsus and flexing the digits. [760- 762]

The forelimb SDFT is considered the most crucial tendon for energy storage and is frequently injured in horses. It is also used as a model for studying Achilles tendon injuries in humans due to its energy-storing capacity, although it has unique anatomical characteristics compared to the human Achilles tendon. [762, 763] The proximal portion of the superficial digital flexor tendon (SDFT) in the forelimb connects the SDFT muscle, which originates from the humerus, to the second phalanx, resulting in flexion of the metacarpophalangeal and proximal interphalangeal joints.

This part of the tendon travels downward along the palmar side of the carpus, passing through the synovial structure of the carpal canal, where it merges with the accessory ligament of the SDFT from the distal radius, before continuing along the palmar aspect of the metacarpus until it reaches the metacarpophalangeal joint.

Around the palmar aspect of the metacarpophalangeal joint, the SDFT encircles the deep digital flexor tendon within the synovial structure of the digital flexor tendon sheath before dividing and attaching to the medial and lateral sides of the second phalanx.

Differences in anatomical structure, such as the elongated length of the equine SDFT and the split insertion points without associated bursae, likely contribute to variations in types of SDFT injuries and their healing potential when compared to injuries in the Achilles tendon and common calcaneal tendon.

Tendon healing is a complex process across all species, often resulting in suboptimal repair tissue formation that is prone to failure and reinjury due to its scar-like composition with increased collagen type III and disorganized fiber patterns, leading to reduced biomechanical strength and elasticity compared to healthy tendon tissue.

Reinjury following midbody or midsubstance tendon injuries is common at the interface between the normal tendon tissue and the scar tissue due to the compromised structure of the scar tissue, making the tendon more vulnerable to future damage.

Tendon healing in cases of tendon ruptures and insertional tendon injuries can be further complicated by factors such as tendon mineralization and adhesions. These complications can lead to a loss of tendon gliding properties, restricted range of motion, and increased pain. Adhesions are a common issue in tendon injuries within synovial structures, often accompanied by synovial inflammation like tenosynovitis or bursitis. Given these challenges, there is a pressing need for innovative therapies aimed at enhancing tendon healing, reducing failure rates, and minimizing reinjury risks.

The objective of this article is to assess the existing evidence supporting the use of mesenchymal stem cells (MSCs) to enhance tendon healing in horses and explore how these findings could be applied to other veterinary species and even humans. [767- 769]

SDFT Core Lesions in Horses

While there exist various forms of injuries to the superficial digital flexor tendon (SDFT) in horses, the most prevalent type is the core lesion in the forelimb. These lesions are commonly found in the extrasynovial midbody of the SDFT in the region between the carpal canal and the digital flexor tendon sheath. Although ruptures and insertional diseases of the SDFT have been documented, they are infrequent occurrences. Forelimb core lesions in the SDFT are more prevalent in horses engaged in activities requiring high speeds, such as racehorses and eventers, but can also affect horses in other disciplines.

Just as a core is pivotal to the structure of a fruit or a core belief is central to one's character, a tendon core lesion is crucial to the integrity of the tendon. While SDFT core lesions may vary in shape and location, they typically encompass a significant portion of the tendon with a rim of unaffected tissue surrounding them, leading to visible lameness. When examined using ultrasonography, the lesion appears hypoechoic, particularly in the initial stages, and the overall cross-sectional area of the SDFT may be notably enlarged due to swelling. This swelling of the SDFT is visible on the underside of the horse's limb and is commonly referred to as a "bowed" tendon due to its appearance.

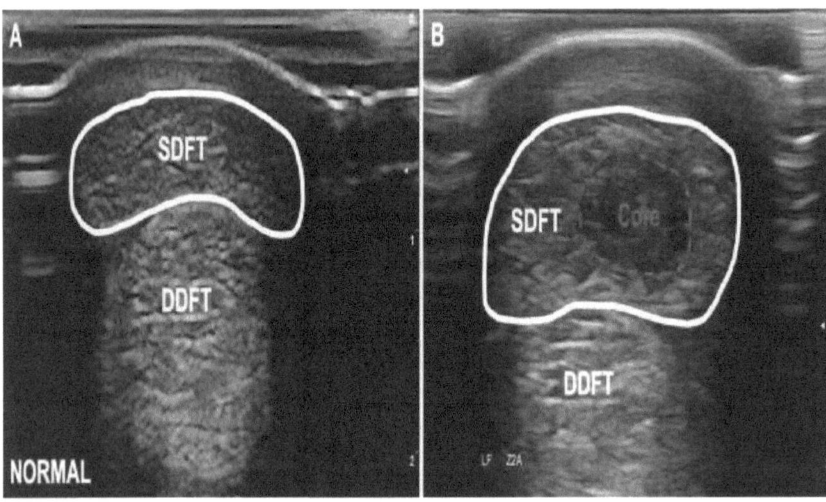

Figure 16

Ultrasound images of the superficial digital flexor tendon (SDFT) in a healthy eventing horse are shown in white (A), in comparison to an enlarged SDFT from another eventing horse, also outlined in white, showcasing a typical hypoechoic core lesion marked in red (B). The deep digital flexor tendon is identified as the DDFT.

Treating core lesions in the suspensory ligament of horses using mesenchymal stem cells

The treatment of core lesions in the superficial digital flexor tendon (SDFT) in horses has significantly progressed over the last two decades, especially in the realm of biologic therapies like stem cells, rehabilitation methods, and controlled exercise regimens. This article aims to specifically explore the use of mesenchymal stem cells (MSCs) for treating core lesions in the SDFT, without delving into other treatment options. Unlike tendon tears and ruptures, core lesions in tendons present a unique opportunity to introduce MSCs into a localized area before the formation of granulation or scar tissue. Although MSCs are not believed to remain in the core lesion for an extended period, they do survive and stay within the lesion in large quantities for at least 10 days, with their viability gradually decreasing over the next 30 to 60 days.[771-773]

For an extended duration, equine professionals have been taking advantage of this opportunity to perform ultrasound-guided intralesional injections of MSCs. These injections are widely accepted as the standard treatment for core lesions in various regions across the globe and are typically reimbursed by insurance for performance horses. The process involves carefully inserting a needle through the healthy tendon perimeter and into the hypoechoic core lesion, as depicted in Figure 7. The introduction of the MSC suspension allows for the visualization of the suspension and any hyperechoic air bubbles within the lesion. Proper sedation of the horse and local anesthesia of the limb using a small-gauge needle (typically size 20 to 23 gauge) is recommended to minimize potential damage to the normal tendon. Even with the use of small-gauge needles, visible needle tracks may persist for a few weeks during subsequent examinations. [774]

There were initial concerns about the impact of needle size on the viability of mesenchymal stem cells (MSCs) after injection. However, research has demonstrated that MSCs can retain their viability when injected through a needle as small as 30 gauge, as long as the injection process involves a single insertion and avoids repeated or rapid aspiration for resuspension.[775, 776]

MSCs should be carefully mixed in the vial they are delivered in, using gentle agitation techniques such as inversion or flicking the bottom of the vial to avoid compromising the sterility of the cap. Prior to injection, MSCs should be aspirated once using a large-gauge needle (20 gauge or larger) before switching to the desired needle size. The ideal timing, dosage, stem cell count per treatment, suitable vehicle for MSC suspension, and frequency of treatments are still awaiting determination.

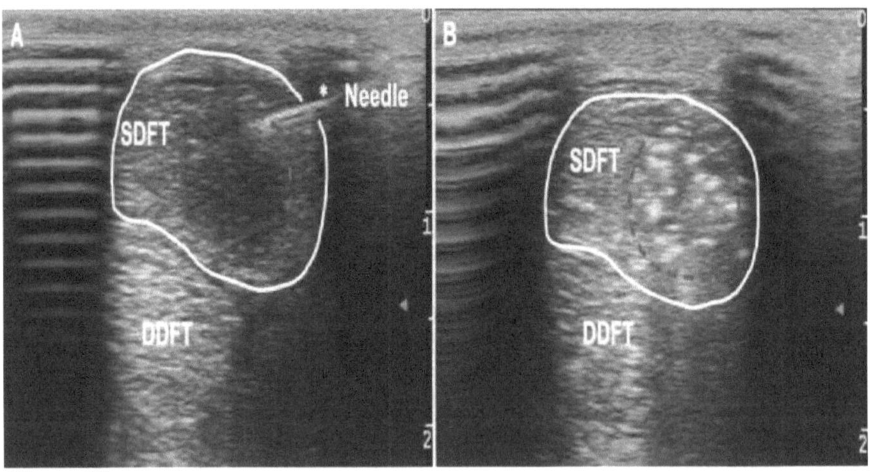

Figure 17

The image presented in Figure 6, panel B, depicts a core lesion in the superficial digital flexor tendon (SDFT) which has been slightly adjusted to facilitate the intralesional injection of mesenchymal stem cells (MSCs) under ultrasound guidance. The first image (A) portrays a hyperechoic needle positioned within the outlined core lesion of the SDFT before injection, while the second image (B) shows the post-injection state with MSCs and hyperechoic air bubbles filling the outlined core lesion. It is worth noting that DDFT refers to the Deep digital flexor tendon.

Over the course of the last two decades of utilizing clinical MSCs in equine treatment, there have been significant lessons learned regarding what practices to avoid. It is crucial to ensure the exclusion of fetal bovine serum (FBS) from the MSC culture medium no less than 48 to 72 hours before cell processing in order to prevent any potential immunological responses to the FBS.[777, 778]

- In many cases, doctors choose to use the patient's own serum rather than fetal bovine serum (FBS) when injecting mesenchymal stem cells (MSCs) into the damaged tissue, with the MSCs being suspended in the same serum. Platelet lysate and other biologics derived from the patient have also been used for this purpose.

- It is important to emphasize that the suspension of MSCs should be kept free from antibiotics or steroids, as the presence of these substances can result in the demise of the MSCs. [780]

Regardless of the type of vehicle being used, it is crucial to recognize that the majority of SDFT core lesions can only accommodate a limited injection volume of less than 1 mL, unless the core lesion stretches from the proximal to distal end. It is essential to discontinue injecting the core lesion once resistance is felt during the injection process, as further delivery of MSC suspension (or any other substance) could result in tendon fiber separation and lesion expansion, potentially leading to increased lameness. The frequency of MSC treatments administered to the patient is mainly determined by the size of the core lesion and the clinician's preference, considering the proper placement of the needle through the normal tendon and the ability to inject an appropriate volume of MSC suspension into the lesion.

In scenarios where the lesion is significantly reduced in size or has been replaced with repair tissue upon reexamination using ultrasound, extra intralesional injections are typically omitted to minimize potential harm to the healthy tendon margin and to prevent excessive injection volume into the lesion. To address any remaining issues at this juncture, if needed, a viable option is the regional limb perfusion of MSCs through either the cephalic vein or the median artery. [781- 783]

A detailed presentation of the decision-making process for treatment and a comprehensive rehabilitation protocol for a standard SDFT core lesion is provided. **(Figure 18)**.

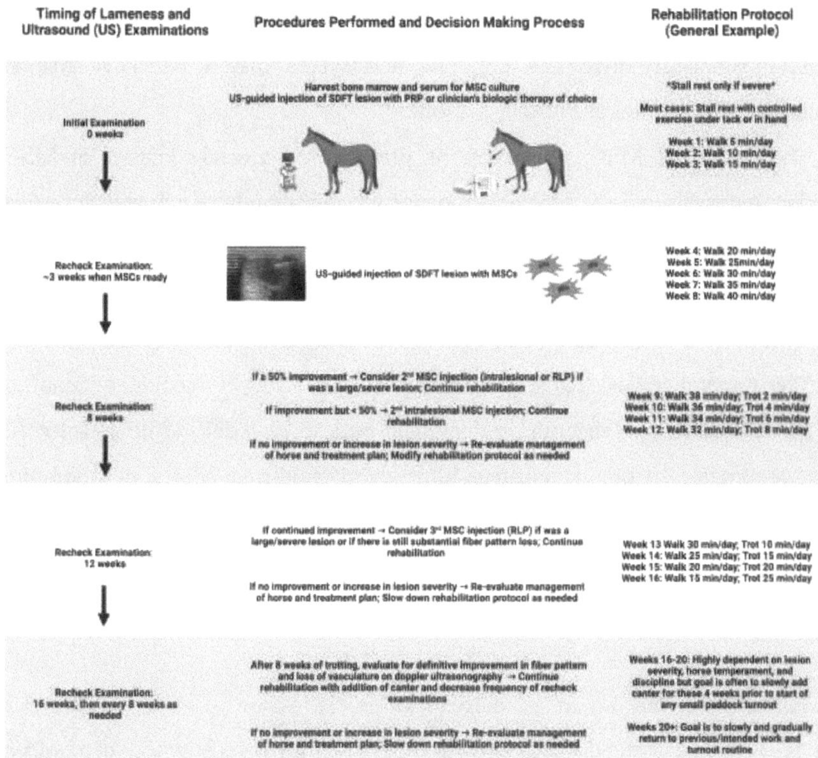

Figure 18

This diagram provides an illustrative depiction of the decision-making process involved in treating a common core lesion of the superficial digital flexor tendon (SDFT) in horses, along with a general rehabilitation protocol. The diagram was generated using BioRender.com. Platelet-rich plasma (PRP) and regional limb perfusion (RLP) are integral components of the treatment plan for this condition.

The ideal timing for the initial administration of MSC therapy presents a compelling query regarding the interaction of MSCs with the site of injury and their reaction to inflammation. Initially thought to have detrimental effects on MSCs, inflammatory cytokines are now believed to play a beneficial role in stimulating MSCs to release healing factors. [784-786]

The notion of MSC stimulation or priming is frequently known as MSC licensing and is discussed in the accompanying publication by Koch and Schnabel in AJVR, October 2023. A recent research project involved the insertion of inert ultrafiltration probes into surgically induced SDFT core lesions in horses in order to analyze the chronological cytokine profile in the core lesions post-injury.[787]

The research revealed that the primary proinflammatory cytokines identified were IL-1β and IL-6, with both reaching their peak levels within 48 hours after the injury occurred. Upon stimulating bone marrow-derived MSCs in laboratory conditions with comparable concentrations of IL-1β or IL-6 obtained from the SDFT core lesions, it was observed that IL-1β triggered the activation of various genes that support tendon healing, as indicated through RNA sequencing analysis. [787].

Furthermore, this led to an increase in the expression of important proteins such as IL-6, vascular endothelial growth factor, and prostaglandin E2, all of which play significant roles in the healing of tendons. These discoveries indicate that the early administration of MSCs for a tendon injury during the acute phase may offer benefits in terms of the natural activation of cells in the body. However, this acute phase is typically brief and may not always be practical in a clinical setting.

One of the current obstacles in utilizing MSCs for treating equine tendon injuries is the precise timing and availability of these cells. The most substantial evidence from both preclinical and clinical studies so far has been seen with autologous bone marrow-derived MSCs. Therefore, the timing for the first MSC treatment is reliant on the diagnosis of the horse and the speed at which bone marrow can be extracted for the preparation of autologous MSC culture, expansion, and injection, a process that usually takes 2 to 3 weeks.

The utility of allogeneic bone marrow-derived MSCs has been acknowledged for several reasons, including the elimination of bone marrow procurement, maintenance of high-quality screened cells readily available for immediate use, and the potential for earlier intervention. Nevertheless, various studies conducted in vitro and in vivo in horses have illustrated immune responses, both cellular and humoral, to major histocompatibility complex (MHC) mismatched bone marrow-derived MSCs, as well as evidence of MSC cytotoxicity in reaction to antibody production. [788- 790]

Efforts are currently being made to regulate the immunogenicity of bone marrow-derived mesenchymal stem cells (MSCs) in the clinical environment, as MHC haplotyping and matching are not feasible. One method being explored involves culturing MSCs with TGF-β2, which has been demonstrated to reduce MHC expression on the surface of MSCs and inhibit MSC cytotoxicity. Furthermore, recent studies have revealed that TGF-β2 can also boost the expression of paracrine factors associated with tendon healing in bone marrow-derived MSCs.[791- 793]

The empirical evidence that validates the application of mesenchymal stem cells for the treatment of tendon core lesions in equines

At present, there have been one minor and two major retrospective clinical trials investigating naturally-occurring forelimb SDFT core lesions, each with long-term follow-up. The results from these studies consistently support the effectiveness of utilizing autologous bone marrow-derived MSCs. [794, 774, 795]

In all three studies, untreated (unlicensed) MSCs were utilized as the exclusive form of therapy. The initial clinical case-controlled series involved 11 flat racehorses treated with autologous bone marrow–derived MSCs, compared to 15 control racehorses from the same practice who received unspecified traditional methods. Both sets of horses underwent the same rehabilitation program. The dosage of administered MSCs varied significantly, ranging from 600,000 to 31.2 million cells, with injections occurring between 18 to 35 days post-injury. Among the MSC-treated group, 9 out of 11 horses (82%) returned to racing within 9 to 12 months and remained free from reinjury at the 2-year mark following MSC treatment. In contrast, all 15 control horses experienced reinjury events within one year, with an average reinjury time of 7 months. Interestingly, the horse that received the lowest number of MSCs was one of the two that did not recover well or return to racing.

In a subsequent extensive clinical study, a cohort of 105 National Hunt horses that participated in racing with jumping underwent treatment with autologous MSCs and supervised rehabilitation. This group was then compared to prior research findings regarding the management of naturally occurring SDFT core lesions in horses. Control horses received alternative treatments such as regulated exercise and medical interventions involving hyaluronan or polysulfated glycosaminoglycans, intralesional injection of IGF-1, and procedures like firing or desmotomy of the accessory (superior/proximal check) ligament of the SDFT. A small number of flat Thoroughbred racehorses were also part of the study; however, the sample size was inadequate for statistical comparison or definitive conclusions. The quantity of MSCs used varied significantly in this study, ranging from a few million to over 50 million, as did the duration between injury and implantation, which varied from approximately 20 days to more than 180 days. Notably, there was a notable decrease in reinjury occurrences among National Hunt horses treated with MSCs (25.7%) compared to those receiving conventional therapies (56% in a previous study and 53% in another). .[774]

There were no significant differences noted in the percentage of National Hunt horses receiving MSC treatment compared to previous data, in relation to their performance in returning to racing and completing 3 and 5 races successfully. An analysis of MSC-treated horses that did not experience reinjury versus those that did showed that the reinjured horses typically received fewer MSCs, were older, and had a longer period between injury and treatment placement, though these differences did not reach statistical significance.

In a recent comprehensive clinical case-control study, a cohort of 213 Thoroughbred flat racehorses with naturally occurring SDFT core lesions were all subjected to the same 12-month controlled exercise rehabilitation regimen. Within this cohort, 66 horses underwent a single treatment of intralesional autologous bone marrow–derived MSCs (10 million cells) around three weeks after the diagnosis of the injury, while 17 horses received a single treatment of intralesional allogeneic adipose-derived MSCs (21 million cells) approximately seven days after the diagnosis. All horses were closely monitored for at least two years after returning to racing. When compared to the outcomes of control horses on a controlled exercise regimen alone, only those treated with autologous bone marrow–derived MSCs showed a significantly higher likelihood of returning to racing (OR, 3.19; 95% CI, 1.55 to 6.81) and completing 5 or more races following the injury (OR, 2.64; 95% CI, 1.32 to 5.33).

In conclusion, the results of these three clinical case series provide support for the effectiveness of utilizing autologous bone marrow-derived mesenchymal stem cells in combination with a closely monitored rehabilitation program for the treatment of core lesions in the superficial digital flexor tendon (SDFT) of horses. The findings demonstrate a greater likelihood of returning to peak performance and a reduced risk of re-injury compared to horses undergoing rehabilitation alone, indicating improved tendon healing that correlates with results from scientific studies conducted prior to clinical trials. These scientific studies have used histological analysis to illustrate enhanced tendon composition, marked by a heightened proportion of type I collagen to type III collagen and more organized tendon structure.

Injuries to the Achilles tendon in both human and canine populations

Upon contemplation of the current understanding regarding the application of MSCs in treating SDFT core lesions in horses, it raises notable inquiries about Achilles tendon injuries in humans and dogs, which may explain the absence of MSC evidence in these species thus far.[796]

In both humans and horses, Achilles tendon injuries are commonly characterized by their chronic and degenerative nature. As such, it is crucial to examine whether these injuries exhibit a similar inflammatory environment to acute core lesions in the superficial digital flexor tendon (SDFT) of horses. There is a possibility that in vitro mesenchymal stem cell (MSC) licensing could play a key role in enhancing treatment outcomes for these injuries, particularly if the MSCs are not receiving the necessary signals from the injury site. Additionally, injuries to the Achilles tendon in both species can present as either noninsertional or insertional, and may involve partial or complete ruptures or avulsions. **(Figure 9).**[756- 761, 767, 797, 798]

The situation outlined here differs significantly from the confined SDFT core lesion in horses, which serves as an optimal site for the delivery and retention of cells, enabling MSCs to interact with the injured tissue environment and release paracrine factors. It remains unclear how long the MSCs stay in proximity to the injury site when injected near the site of rupture or avulsion, and the extent of their interaction with the damaged tendon environment. Given this scenario, the question arises whether MSCs should be administered in a gel or on a scaffold to enhance retention. The concept of MSCs or MSC-secreted factors diffusing out of the calcaneal bursa to reach the injured tendon presents an intriguing area that calls for further investigation. Additionally, in the context of insertional tendinopathies, a consideration arises as to whether MSCs should be directed towards promoting the production of type II and type X collagen, which are specifically found in the tendon at that insertion site. It is imperative to conduct further research in this domain, as MSC licensing may offer a innovative approach for the precise treatment of tendon injuries based on location and type.

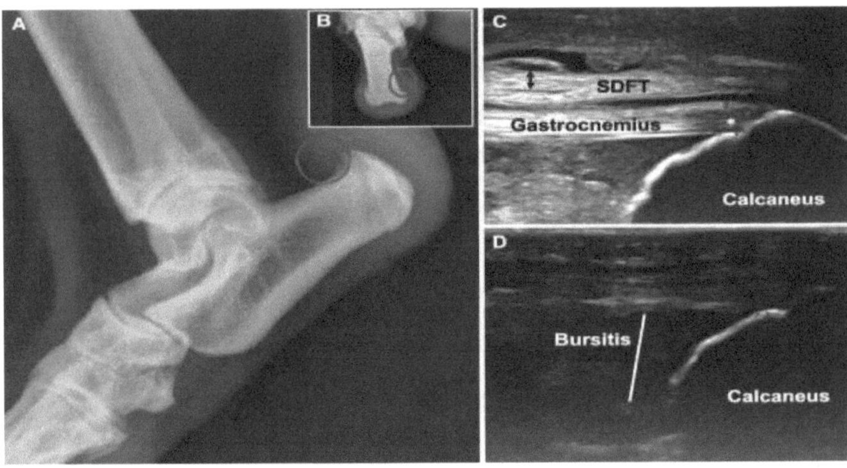

Figure 19

Example lateral (A) and skyline (B) radiographs along with sagittal plane ultrasound images (C and D) of the tarsus in a German Shorthair Pointer hunting dog exhibit a prevalent calcaneal tendon (CCT) injury. Anomalies such as dystrophic mineralization and/or avulsion fragments are noticeable in close proximity to the insertion point of the CCT on the calcaneus, as highlighted by the red circles on the radiographs (A and B). The ultrasound images unveil signs of tears in the superficial digital flexor tendon (SDFT) as indicated by the arrows, in addition to a widespread tendonitis, alterations in the fiber pattern of the gastrocnemius tendon at the insertion on the calcaneus implicative of partial rupture (asterisk), and calcaneal bursitis (D).

Conclusion

Veterinary regenerative medicine is an evolving area of research, marked by significant advancements in the development of safe and effective stem cell therapies in recent years. Encouraging results have been seen in the use of mesenchymal stem cell (MSC) therapies for orthopedic conditions in dogs and horses, as well as in addressing conditions like FCGS, IBD, and wound healing. Numerous studies have shown promising outcomes for stem cell therapies in animal diseases, suggesting a bright future ahead. However, there are key challenges that remain to be overcome, such as identifying the optimal source for MSC isolation. Although adipose and bone marrow derived MSCs are commonly used due to their accessibility and ease of use, stem cells from different tissues may offer improved efficacy in treating specific diseases in the future.

Moreover, additional studies are required to gain insight into how factors like age and gender affect the therapeutic efficacy of MSCs. Discrepancies in disease development, cell quantity, and techniques for administering MSCs in various research studies underscore the absence of uniform protocols for the most effective treatment regimens. Despite worries surrounding the short lifespan and quick elimination of cells, the intravenous delivery of MSCs continues to be a widely accepted method for addressing a range of animal illnesses.

However, as per some research, it has been suggested that immune cells in the body can initiate healing processes through apoptosis-mediated immunomodulation, which may enhance the benefits of MSC therapy. The challenge lies in the fact that MSCs tend to remain in the lungs after being administered intravenously, which hinders their effectiveness in systemic stem cell treatments. Despite efforts to find other ways to avoid this lung entrapment issue, systemic administration of ECV has emerged as a leading alternative to intravenous MSC infusion.

Preliminary investigations suggest that extracellular vesicles (ECVs) show potential as a stem cell therapy devoid of cells, which could help alleviate lung entrapment and lower the risk of pulmonary embolism linked to the intravenous administration of mesenchymal stem cells (MSCs). However, additional research is needed to assess the effectiveness and safety of ECVs. The decision between using autologous and allogeneic cells remains undecided. Although autologous cells are considered safer, their application is more complex and costly for pet owners. Allogeneic cells from healthy donors offer a viable option, although concerns persist regarding their immunogenicity and potential to induce an immune response in recipients.

Despite the considerable progress made in recent years in the field of veterinary regenerative medicine, there is still much to be discovered and researched before well-established treatments can be made available to patients. The current era is characterized by the rapid advancement of regenerative therapies, offering hope for the future of stem cell treatments in both veterinary and human medicine. Ongoing studies are continuously being conducted in the realm of regenerative medicine for animals. Recent years have seen significant advancements in the development of safe and effective stem cell therapies. Notable progress has been made in MSC therapy, particularly for conditions like FCGS, IBD, and wound healing, showing promising results in orthopedic issues in dogs and horses. Research has demonstrated positive outcomes, indicating the potential of stem cell therapy for a wide array of animal diseases in the future. However, there are still various challenges that need to be addressed.

Identifying the most suitable source for isolating MSCs presents a considerable challenge. At present, researchers commonly rely on MSCs obtained from adipose tissue and bone marrow due to their convenience and manageability. There is speculation that stem cells from alternative organs may prove more effective in addressing certain medical conditions in the future. Furthermore, additional investigations are required to understand the influence of age and potentially gender on the therapeutic potential of MSCs. Discrepancies in findings persist across various studies concerning disease advancement, cell quantity, and modes of administration.

A standardized protocol for determining the most effective treatments for specific conditions has not yet been developed. Despite concerns about the short lifespan and quick elimination of cells, the intravenous administration of MSCs has been widely used in treating various animal diseases. Some research suggests that the immunomodulation triggered by apoptosis in immune cells could stimulate the body's natural healing mechanisms, potentially extending the benefits of MSC therapy.

One of the main challenges in systemic stem cell treatments is retaining MSCs in the lungs after intravenous administration. An alternative to intravenous delivery of MSCs is the systemic administration of ECVs, with different methods being explored to prevent lung entrapment. Initial studies indicate that ECVs could offer a promising cell-free therapy to reduce lung entrapment and lower the risk of pulmonary embolism following intravenous MSC injections, although further research is necessary to assess the safety and efficacy of ECVs. The use of autologous or allogeneic cells presents an unresolved dilemma, as while autologous cells are deemed safer, they present logistical and financial challenges for animal owners. Therefore, allogeneic cells from healthy donors are viewed as a practical alternative, even though concerns exist about their potential immunogenicity and ability to provoke an immune response in recipients.

The field of veterinary regenerative medicine has made notable progress, yet it is still in its preliminary phases and requires ongoing dedication to resolve various challenges before standardized treatments can be provided to patients. The present state of regenerative medicine offers hope for the creation of groundbreaking therapies that could play a key role in addressing numerous untreatable illnesses in both veterinary and human healthcare. Continued research is expected to solidify stem cell therapies as a powerful treatment choice, rather than merely a hypothetical idea.

Improving in vitro biomedical models is essential for the progression of medical research. Significant progress has been made in organoid research, especially in the realm of rodent organoids for investigating the genetic basis of diseases. Despite various advancements, the ability to apply these models to different areas is still restricted. By harnessing the varied qualities found in the animal kingdom, there is potential for further advancements in both biomedical and translational research. Animal-based organoids, such as those from canines, offer distinctive opportunities for facilitating the exchange of knowledge between human and veterinary medicine through a reverse translational method.

References

1. Morrison SJ, Wandycz AM, Hemmati HD, Wright DE, Weissman IL. Identification of a lineage of multipotent hematopoietic progenitors. *Development*. (1997) 124:1929–39.
2. Evans MJ, Kaufman MH. Establishment in culture of pluripotential cells from mouse embryos. *Nature*. (1981) 292:154–6. doi: 10.1038/292154a0
3. Takahashi K, Yamanaka S. Induction of pluripotent stem cells from mouse embryonic and adult fibroblast cultures by defined factors. *Cell*. (2006) 126:663–76. doi: 10.1016/j.cell.2006.07.024
4. Wagers AJ, Weissman IL. Plasticity of adult stem cells. *Cell*. (2004) 116:639–48. doi: 10.1016/S0092-8674(04)00208-9
5. Martin GR. Isolation of a pluripotent cell line from early mouse embryos cultured in medium conditioned by teratocarcinoma stem cells. *Proc Natl Acad Sci USA*. (1981) 78:7634–8. doi: 10.1073/pnas.78.12.7634
6. Thomson JA, Marshall VS. Primate embryonic stem cells. *Curr Top Dev Biol*. (1998) 38:133–65. doi: 10.1016/S0070-2153(08)60246-X
7. Thomson JA, Itskovitz-Eldor J, Shapiro SS, Waknitz MA, Swiergiel JJ, Marshall VS, et al. Embryonic stem cell lines derived from human blastocysts. *Science*. (1998) 282:1145–7. doi: 10.1126/science.282.5391.1145
8. Caplan AI. Mesenchymal stem cells. *J Orthop Res*. (1991) 9:641–50. doi: 10.1002/jor.1100090504
9. Friedenstein AJ, Petrakova KV, Kurolesova AI, Frolova GP. Heterotopic of bone marrow. Analysis of precursor cells for osteogenic and hematopoietic tissues. *Transplantation*. (1968) 6:230–47. doi: 10.1097/00007890-196803000-00009

10. Dennis JE, Merriam A, Awadallah A, Yoo JU, Johnstone B, Caplan AI. A quadripotential mesenchymal progenitor cell isolated from the marrow of an adult mouse. *J Bone Miner Res*. (1999) 14:700–9. doi: 10.1359/jbmr.1999.14.5.700
11. Miyahara Y, Nagaya N, Kataoka M, Yanagawa B, Tanaka K, Hao H, et al. Monolayered mesenchymal stem cells repair scarred myocardium after myocardial infarction. *Nat Med*. (2006) 12:459–65. doi: 10.1038/nm1391
12. Quinn C, Flake AW. *In vivo* differentiation potential of mesenchymal stem cells: prenatal and postnatal model systems. *Transfus Med Hemother*. (2008) 35:239–47. doi: 10.1159/000129129
13. Niess H, Thomas MN, Schiergens TS, Kleespies A, Jauch KW, Bruns C, et al. Genetic engineering of mesenchymal stromal cells for cancer therapy: turning partners in crime into Trojan horses. *Innov Surg Sci*. (2016) 1:19–32. doi: 10.1515/iss-2016-0005
14. Caplan AI. Mesenchymal stem cells: time to change the name! stem cells. *Transl Med.* (2017). 6:1445–51. doi: 10.1002/sctm.17-0051
15. Dominici M, Le Blanc K, Mueller I, Slaper-Cortenbach I, Marini F, Krause D, et al. Minimal criteria for defining multipotent mesenchymal stromal cells. The international society for cellular therapy position statement. *Cytotherapy*. (2006) 8:315–7. doi: 10.1080/14653240600855905
16. Sasaki A, Mizuno M, Ozeki N, Katano H, Otabe K, Tsuji K, et al. Canine mesenchymal stem cells from synovium have a higher chondrogenic potential than those from infrapatellar fat pad, adipose tissue, and bone marrow. *PLoS ONE*. (2018) 13:e0202922. doi: 10.1371/journal.pone.0202922
17. Bearden RN, Huggins SS, Cummings KJ, Smith R, Gregory CA, Saunders WB. In-vitro characterization of canine multipotent stromal cells isolated

from synovium, bone marrow, and adipose tissue: a donor-matched comparative study. *Stem Cell Res Ther*. (2017) 8:218. doi: 10.1186/s13287-017-0639-6

18. Zhang S, Zhao C, Liu S, Wang Y, Zhao Y, Guan W, et al. Characteristics and multilineage differentiation of bone marrow mesenchymal stem cells derived from the Tibetan mastiff. *Mol Med Rep*. (2018) 18:2097–109. doi: 10.3892/mmr.2018.9172
19. Kang BJ, Ryu HH, Park SS, Koyama Y, Kikuchi M, Woo HM, et al. Comparing the osteogenic potential of canine mesenchymal stem cells derived from adipose tissues, bone marrow, umbilical cord blood, and Wharton's Jelly for treating bone defects. *J Vet Sci*. (2012) 13:299–310. doi: 10.4142/jvs.2012.13.3.299
20. Radtke CL, Nino-Fong R, Esparza, Gonzalez BP, Stryhn H, McDuffee LA. Characterization and osteogenic potential of equine muscle tissue- and periosteal tissue-derived mesenchymal stem cells in comparison with bone marrow- and adipose tissue-derived mesenchymal stem cells. *Am J Vet Res*. (2013) 74:790–800. doi: 10.2460/ajvr.74.5.790
21. Arevalo-Turrubiarte M, Olmeo C, Accornero P, Baratta M, Martignani E. Analysis of mesenchymal cells (MSCs) from bone marrow, synovial fluid and mesenteric, neck and tail adipose tissue sources from equines. *Stem Cell Res*. (2019) 37:101442. doi: 10.1016/j.scr.2019.101442
22. Martin DR, Cox NR, Hathcock TL, Niemeyer GP, Baker HJ. Isolation and characterization of multipotential mesenchymal stem cells from feline bone marrow. *Exp Hematol*. (2002) 30:879–86. doi: 10.1016/S0301-472X(02)00864-0

23. Webb TL, Quimby JM, Dow SW. *In vitro* comparison of feline bone marrow-derived and adipose tissue-derived mesenchymal stem cells. *J Feline Med Surg*. (2012) 14:165–8. doi: 10.1177/1098612X11429224
24. Lee BY, Li Q, Song WJ, Chae HK, Kweon K, Ahn JO, et al. Altered properties of feline adipose-derived mesenchymal stem cells during continuous *in vitro* cultivation. *J Vet Med Sci*. (2018) 80:930–8. doi: 10.1292/jvms.17-0563
25. Krawetz RJ, Wu YE, Martin L, Rattner JB, Matyas JR, Hart DA. Synovial fluid progenitors expressing CD90+ from normal but not osteoarthritic joints undergo chondrogenic differentiation without micro-mass culture. *PLoS ONE*. (2012) 7:e43616. doi: 10.1371/journal.pone.0043616
26. Prado AA, Favaron PO, da Silva LC, Baccarin RY, Miglino MA, Maria DA. Characterization of mesenchymal stem cells derived from the equine synovial fluid and membrane. *BMC Vet Res*. (2015) 11:281. doi: 10.1186/s12917-015-0531-5
27. Zhang BY, Wang BY, Li SC, Luo DZ, Zhan X, Chen SF, et al. Evaluation of the curative effect of umbilical cord mesenchymal stem cell therapy for knee arthritis in dogs using imaging technology. *Stem Cells Int*. (2018) 2018:1983025. doi: 10.1155/2018/1983025
28. Denys M, Leon A, Robert C, Saulnier N, Josson-Schramme A, Legrand L, et al. Biosafety evaluation of equine umbilical cord-derived mesenchymal stromal cells (UC-MSCs) by systematic pathogen screening in peripheral maternal blood and paired UC-MSCs. *Biopreserv Biobank*. (2020) 18:73–81. doi: 10.1089/bio.2019.0071
29. Carrade DD, Affolter VK, Outerbridge CA, Watson JL, Galuppo LD, Buerchler S, et al. Intradermal injections of equine allogeneic umbilical cord-

derived mesenchymal stem cells are well tolerated and do not elicit immediate or delayed hypersensitivity reactions. *Cytotherapy.* (2011) 13:1180–92. doi: 10.3109/14653249.2011.602338

30. Koch TG, Heerkens T, Thomsen PD, Betts DH. Isolation of mesenchymal stem cells from equine umbilical cord blood. *BMC Biotechnol.* (2007) 7:26. doi: 10.1186/1472-6750-7-26
31. Carrade DD, Owens SD, Galuppo LD, Vidal MA, Ferraro GL, Librach F, et al. Clinicopathologic findings following intra-articular injection of autologous and allogeneic placentally derived equine mesenchymal stem cells in horses. *Cytotherapy.* (2011) 13:419–30. doi: 10.3109/14653249.2010.536213
32. Kisiel AH, McDuffee LA, Masaoud E, Bailey TR, Esparza Gonzalez BP, Nino-Fong R. Isolation, characterization, and *in vitro* proliferation of canine mesenchymal stem cells derived from bone marrow, adipose tissue, muscle, and periosteum. *Am J Vet Res.* (2012) 73:1305–17. doi: 10.2460/ajvr.73.8.1305
33. Mensing N, Gasse H, Hambruch N, Haeger JD, Pfarrer C, Staszyk C. Isolation and characterization of multipotent mesenchymal stromal cells from the gingiva and the periodontal ligament of the horse. *BMC Vet Res.* (2011) 7:42. doi: 10.1186/1746-6148-7-42
34. Sato K, Yamawaki-Ogata A, Kanemoto I, Usui A, Narita Y. Isolation and characterisation of peripheral blood-derived feline mesenchymal stem cells. *Vet J.* (2016) 216:183–8. doi: 10.1016/j.tvjl.2016.08.009
35. Longhini ALF, Salazar TE, Vieira C, Trinh T, Duan Y, Pay LM, et al. Peripheral blood-derived mesenchymal stem cells demonstrate immunomodulatory potential for therapeutic use in horses. *PLoS ONE.* (2019) 14:e0212642. doi: 10.1371/journal.pone.0212642

36. Spaas JH, Broeckx S, Van de Walle GR, Polettini M. The effects of equine peripheral blood stem cells on cutaneous wound healing: a clinical evaluation in four horses. *Clin Exp Dermatol*. (2013) 38:280–4. doi: 10.1111/ced.12068
37. Marfe G, Massaro-Giordano M, Ranalli M, Cozzoli E, Di Stefano C, Malafoglia V, et al. Blood derived stem cells: an ameliorative therapy in veterinary ophthalmology. *J Cell Physiol*. (2012) 227:1250–6. doi: 10.1002/jcp.22953
38. Rink BE, Amilon KR, Esteves CL, French HM, Watson E, Aurich C, et al. Isolation and characterization of equine endometrial mesenchymal stromal cells. *Stem Cell Res Ther*. (2017) 8:166. doi: 10.1186/s13287-017-0616-0
39. da Silva Meirelles L, Chagastelles PC, Nardi NB. Mesenchymal stem cells reside in virtually all post-natal organs and tissues. *J Cell Sci*. (2006) 119:2204–13. doi: 10.1242/jcs.02932
40. Russell KA, Chow NH, Dukoff D, Gibson TW, LaMarre J, Betts DH, et al. Characterization and immunomodulatory effects of canine adipose tissue- and bone marrow-derived mesenchymal stromal cells. *PLoS ONE*. (2016) 11:e0167442. doi: 10.1371/journal.pone.0167442
41. Villatoro AJ, Alcoholado C, Martin-Astorga MC, Fernandez V, Cifuentes M, Becerra J. Comparative analysis and characterization of soluble factors and exosomes from cultured adipose tissue and bone marrow mesenchymal stem cells in canine species. *Vet Immunol Immunopathol*. (2019) 208:6–15. doi: 10.1016/j.vetimm.2018.12.003
42. Vidal MA, Robinson SO, Lopez MJ, Paulsen DB, Borkhsenious O, Johnson JR, et al. Comparison of chondrogenic potential in equine mesenchymal stromal cells derived from adipose tissue and bone marrow. *Vet Surg*. (2008) 37:713–24. doi: 10.1111/j.1532-950X.2008.00462.x

43. Fideles SOM, Ortiz AC, Assis AF, Duarte MJ, Oliveira FS, Passos GA, et al. Effect of cell source and osteoblast differentiation on gene expression profiles of mesenchymal stem cells derived from bone marrow or adipose tissue. *J Cell Biochem*. (2019) 120: 11842–52. doi: 10.1002/jcb.28463
44. Guercio A, Di Bella S, Casella S, Di Marco P, Russo C, Piccione G. Canine mesenchymal stem cells (MSCs): characterization in relation to donor age and adipose tissue-harvesting site. *Cell Biol Int*. (2013) 37:789–98. doi: 10.1002/cbin.10090
45. Yaneselli KM, Kuhl CP, Terraciano PB, de Oliveira FS, Pizzato SB, Pazza K, et al. Comparison of the characteristics of canine adipose tissue-derived mesenchymal stem cells extracted from different sites and at different passage numbers. *J Vet Sci*. (2018) 19:13–20. doi: 10.4142/jvs.2018.19.1.13
46. Bahamondes F, Flores E, Cattaneo G, Bruna F, Conget P. Omental adipose tissue is a more suitable source of canine mesenchymal stem cells. *BMC Vet Res*. (2017) 13:166. doi: 10.1186/s12917-017-1053-0
47. Boxall SA, Jones E. Markers for characterization of bone marrow multipotential stromal cells. *Stem Cells Int*. (2012) 2012:975871. doi: 10.1155/2012/975871
48. FDA. *CVMGFI #218 Cell-Based Products for Animal Use.* (2015). Available online at: https://www.fda.gov/media/88925/download (accessed February 15, 2020).
49. Sancak IG, Ozen A, Bayraktaroglu AG, Ceylan A, Can P. Characterization of mesenchymal stem cells isolated from the adipose tissue of young and old dogs. *Veteriner Fakültesi dergisi*. (2016) 63:297–302. doi: 10.1501/Vetfak_0000002743

50. Zajic B, Webb LT, Webb P, Coy WJ, Quimby MJ. Comparison of proliferative and immunomodulatory potential of adipose-derived mesenchymal stem cells from young and geriatric cats. *J Feline Med Surg*. (2017) 19:1096–102. doi: 10.1177/1098612X16680703
51. Taguchi T, Borjesson DL, Osmond C, Griffon DJ. Influence of donor's age on immunomodulatory properties of canine adipose tissue-derived mesenchymal stem cells. *Stem Cells Dev*. (2019) 28:1562–71. doi: 10.1089/scd.2019.0118
52. Iohara K, Murakami M, Nakata K, Nakashima M. Age-dependent decline in dental pulp regeneration after pulpectomy in dogs. *Exp Gerontol*. (2014) 52:39–45. doi: 10.1016/j.exger.2014.01.020
53. Lee J, Lee KS, Kim CL, Byeon JS, Gu NY, Cho IS, et al. Effect of donor age on the proliferation and multipotency of canine adipose-derived mesenchymal stem cells. *J Vet Sci*. (2017) 18:141–8. doi: 10.4142/jvs.2017.18.2.141
54. Marycz K, Kornicka K, Maredziak M, Golonka P, Nicpon J. Equine metabolic syndrome impairs adipose stem cells osteogenic differentiation by predominance of autophagy over selective mitophagy. *J Cell Mol Med*. (2016) 20:2384–404. doi: 10.1111/jcmm.12932
55. Wieczorek M, Abualrous ET, Sticht J, Alvaro-Benito M, Stolzenberg S, Noe F, et al. Major histocompatibility complex (MHC) class I and MHC class II proteins: conformational plasticity in antigen presentation. *Front Immunol*. (2017) 8:292. doi: 10.3389/fimmu.2017.00292
56. Schnabel LV, Pezzanite LM, Antczak DF, Felippe JB, Fortier LA. Equine bone marrow-derived mesenchymal stromal cells are heterogeneous in MHC class II expression and capable of inciting an immune response *in vitro*. *Stem Cell Res Ther*. (2014) 5:13. doi: 10.1186/scrt402

57. Berglund AK, Schnabel LV. Allogeneic major histocompatibility complex-mismatched equine bone marrow-derived mesenchymal stem cells are targeted for death by cytotoxic anti-major histocompatibility complex antibodies. *Equine Vet J.* (2017) 49:539–44. doi: 10.1111/evj.12647
58. Oliveira RL, Chagastelles PC, Sesterheim P, Pranke P. *In vivo* immunogenic response to allogeneic mesenchymal stem cells and the role of preactivated mesenchymal stem cells cotransplanted with allogeneic islets. *Stem Cells Int.* (2017) 2017:9824698. doi: 10.1155/2017/9824698
59. Ryan AE, Lohan P, O'Flynn L, Treacy O, Chen X, Coleman C, et al. Chondrogenic differentiation increases antidonor immune response to allogeneic mesenchymal stem cell transplantation. *Mol Ther.* (2014) 22:655–67. doi: 10.1038/mt.2013.261
60. Joswig AJ, Mitchell A, Cummings KJ, Levine GJ, Gregory CA, Smith R, et al. Repeated intra-articular injection of allogeneic mesenchymal stem cells causes an adverse response compared to autologous cells in the equine model. *Stem Cell Res Ther.* (2017) 8:42. doi: 10.1186/s13287-017-0503-8
61. Pezzanite LM, Fortier LA, Antczak DF, Cassano JM, Brosnahan MM, Miller D, et al. Equine allogeneic bone marrow-derived mesenchymal stromal cells elicit antibody responses *in vivo*. *Stem Cell Res Ther.* (2015) 6:54. doi: 10.1186/s13287-015-0053-x
62. Ursini TL, Amelse LL, Elkhenany HA, Odoi A, Carter-Arnold JL, Adair HS, et al. Retrospective analysis of local injection site adverse reactions associated with 230 allogenic administrations of bone marrow-derived mesenchymal stem cells in 164 horses. *Equine Vet J.* (2019) 51:198–205. doi: 10.1111/evj.12992

63. Cabon Q, Febre M, Gomez N, Cachon T, Pillard P, Carozzo C, et al. Long-term safety and efficacy of single or repeated intra-articular injection of allogeneic neonatal mesenchymal stromal cells for managing pain and lameness in moderate to severe canine osteoarthritis without anti-inflammatory pharmacological support: pilot clinical study. *Front Vet Sci.* (2019) 6:10. doi: 10.3389/fvets.2019.00010
64. Bertoni L, Branly T, Jacquet S, Desance M, Desquilbet L, Rivory P, et al. Intra-articular injection of 2 different dosages of autologous and allogeneic bone marrow- and umbilical cord-derived mesenchymal stem cells triggers a variable inflammatory response of the fetlock joint on 12 sound experimental horses. *Stem Cells Int*. (2019) 2019:9431894. doi: 10.1155/2019/9431894
65. Magri C, Schramme M, Febre M, Cauvin E, Labadie F, Saulnier N, et al. Comparison of efficacy and safety of single versus repeated intra-articular injection of allogeneic neonatal mesenchymal stem cells for treatment of osteoarthritis of the metacarpophalangeal/metatarsophalangeal joint in horses: a clinical pilot study. *PLoS ONE*. (2019) 14:e0221317. doi: 10.1371/journal.pone.0221317
66. Menard C, Dulong J, Roulois D, Hebraud B, Verdiere L, Pangault C, et al. Integrated transcriptomic, phenotypic, and functional study reveals tissue-specific immune properties of mesenchymal stromal cells. *Stem Cells*. (2019) 38:146–59. doi: 10.1002/stem.3077
67. Souza-Moreira L, Soares VC, Dias S, Bozza PT. Adipose-derived mesenchymal stromal cells modulate lipid metabolism and lipid droplet biogenesis via AKT/mTOR -PPARγ signalling in macrophages. *Sci Rep*. (2019) 9:20304. doi: 10.1038/s41598-019-56835-8

68. Gao WX, Sun YQ, Shi J, Li CL, Fang SB, Wang D, et al. Effects of mesenchymal stem cells from human induced pluripotent stem cells on differentiation, maturation, and function of dendritic cells. *Stem Cell Res Ther*. (2017) 8:48. doi: 10.1186/s13287-017-0499-0
69. Laing AG, Fanelli G, Ramirez-Valdez A, Lechler RI, Lombardi G, Sharpe PT. Mesenchymal stem cells inhibit T-cell function through conserved induction of cellular stress. *PLoS ONE*. (2019) 14:e0213170. doi: 10.1371/journal.pone.0213170
70. Luk F, Carreras-Planella L, Korevaar SS, de Witte SFH, Borras FE, Betjes MGH, et al. Inflammatory conditions dictate the effect of mesenchymal stem or stromal cells on B cell function. *Front Immunol*. (2017) 8:1042. doi: 10.3389/fimmu.2017.01042
71. Spaggiari GM, Capobianco A, Becchetti S, Mingari MC, Moretta L. Mesenchymal stem cell-natural killer cell interactions: evidence that activated NK cells are capable of killing MSCs, whereas MSCs can inhibit IL-2-induced NK-cell proliferation. *Blood*. (2006) 107:1484–90. doi: 10.1182/blood-2005-07-2775
72. Blobe GC, Schiemann WP, Lodish HF. Role of transforming growth factor beta in human disease. *N Engl J Med*. (2000) 342:1350–8. doi: 10.1056/NEJM200005043421807
73. Deng M, Mei T, Hou T, Luo K, Luo F, Yang A, et al. TGFβ3 recruits endogenous mesenchymal stem cells to initiate bone regeneration. *Stem Cell Res Ther*. (2017) 8:258. doi: 10.1186/s13287-017-0693-0
74. Dubon MJ, Yu J, Choi S, Park KS. Transforming growth factor beta induces bone marrow mesenchymal stem cell migration via noncanonical signals and N-cadherin. *J Cell Physiol*. (2018) 233:201–13. doi: 10.1002/jcp.25863

75. Liu F, Qiu H, Xue M, Zhang S, Zhang X, Xu J, et al. MSC-secreted TGF-β regulates lipopolysaccharide-stimulated macrophage M2-like polarization via the Akt/FoxO1 pathway. *Stem Cell Res Ther*. (2019) 10:345. doi: 10.1186/s13287-019-1447-y
76. Wu R, Liu C, Deng X, Chen L, Hao S, Ma L. Enhanced alleviation of aGVHD by TGF-β1-modified mesenchymal stem cells in mice through shifting MPhi into M2 phenotype and promoting the differentiation of Treg cells. *J Cell Mol Med*. (2020) 24:1684–99. doi: 10.1111/jcmm.14862
77. Gazdic M, Markovic BS, Arsenijevic A, Jovicic N, Acovic A, Harrell CR, et al. Crosstalk between mesenchymal stem cells and T regulatory cells is crucially important for the attenuation of acute liver injury. *Liver Transpl*. (2018) 24:687–702. doi: 10.1002/lt.25049
78. Schmidt A, Zhang XM, Joshi RN, Iqbal S, Wahlund C, Gabrielsson S, et al. Human macrophages induce CD4(+)Foxp3(+) regulatory T cells via binding and re-release of TGF-β. *Immunol Cell Biol*. (2016) 94:747–62. doi: 10.1038/icb.2016.34
79. Melief SM, Schrama E, Brugman MH, Tiemessen MM, Hoogduijn MJ, Fibbe WE, et al. Multipotent stromal cells induce human regulatory T cells through a novel pathway involving skewing of monocytes toward anti-inflammatory macrophages. *Stem Cells*. (2013) 31:1980–91. doi: 10.1002/stem.1432
80. Franquesa M, Mensah FK, Huizinga R, Strini T, Boon L, Lombardo E, et al. Human adipose tissue-derived mesenchymal stem cells abrogate plasmablast formation and induce regulatory B cells independently of T helper cells. *Stem Cells*. (2015) 33:880–91. doi: 10.1002/stem.1881
81. Fallarino F, Grohmann U, You S, McGrath BC, Cavener DR, Vacca C, et al. The combined effects of tryptophan starvation and tryptophan catabolites

down-regulate T cell receptor zeta-chain and induce a regulatory phenotype in naive T cells. *J Immunol.* (2006) 176:6752–61. doi: 10.4049/jimmunol.176.11.6752

82. Spaggiari GM, Capobianco A, Abdelrazik H, Becchetti F, Mingari MC, Moretta L. Mesenchymal stem cells inhibit natural killer-cell proliferation, cytotoxicity, and cytokine production: role of indoleamine 2,3-dioxygenase and prostaglandin E2. *Blood.* (2008) 111:1327–33. doi: 10.1182/blood-2007-02-074997
83. Francois M, Romieu-Mourez R, Li M, Galipeau J. Human MSC suppression correlates with cytokine induction of indoleamine 2,3-dioxygenase and bystander M2 macrophage differentiation. *Mol Ther.* (2012) 20:187–95. doi: 10.1038/mt.2011.189
84. Kalinski P. Regulation of immune responses by prostaglandin E2. *J Immunol.* (2012) 188:21–8. doi: 10.4049/jimmunol.1101029
85. Jin L, Deng Z, Zhang J, Yang C, Liu J, Han W, et al. Mesenchymal stem cells promote type 2 macrophage polarization to ameliorate the myocardial injury caused by diabetic cardiomyopathy. *J Transl Med.* (2019) 17:251. doi: 10.1186/s12967-019-1999-8
86. Zhang Z, Huang S, Wu S, Qi J, Li W, Liu S, et al. Clearance of apoptotic cells by mesenchymal stem cells contributes to immunosuppression via PGE2. *EBioMedicine.* (2019) 45:341–50. doi: 10.1016/j.ebiom.2019.06.016
87. de Vries JE. Immunosuppressive and anti-inflammatory properties of interleukin 10. *Ann Med.* (1995) 27:537–41. doi: 10.3109/07853899509002465

88. Couper KN, Blount DG, Riley EM. IL-10: the master regulator of immunity to infection. *J Immunol.* (2008) 180:5771–7. doi: 10.4049/jimmunol.180.9.5771
89. Najar M, Raicevic G, Fayyad-Kazan H, De Bruyn C, Bron D, Toungouz M, et al. Bone marrow mesenchymal stromal cells induce proliferative, cytokinic and molecular changes during the T cell response: the importance of the IL-10/CD210 axis. *Stem Cell Rev Rep*. (2015) 11:442–52. doi: 10.1007/s12015-014-9567-3
90. Day AJ, Milner CM. TSG-6: a multifunctional protein with anti-inflammatory and tissue-protective properties. *Matrix Biol.* (2019) 78–9:60–83. doi: 10.1016/j.matbio.2018.01.011
91. Romano B, Elangovan S, Erreni M, Sala E, Petti L, Kunderfranco P, et al. TNF-stimulated gene-6 is a key regulator in switching stemness and biological properties of mesenchymal stem cells. *Stem Cells*. (2019) 37:973–87. doi: 10.1002/stem.3010
92. An JH, Li Q, Bhang DH, Song WJ, Youn HY. TNF-α and INF-γ primed canine stem cell-derived extracellular vesicles alleviate experimental murine colitis. *Sci Rep*. (2020) 10:2115. doi: 10.1038/s41598-020-58909-4
93. Song WJ, Li Q, Ryu MO, Ahn JO, Bhang DH, Jung YC, et al. TSG-6 released from intraperitoneally injected canine adipose tissue-derived mesenchymal stem cells ameliorate inflammatory bowel disease by inducing M2 macrophage switch in mice. *Stem Cell Res Ther*. (2018) 9:91. doi: 10.1186/s13287-018-0841-1
94. Wang S, Lee JS, Hyun J, Kim J, Kim SU, Cha HJ, et al. Tumor necrosis factor-inducible gene 6 promotes liver regeneration in mice with acute liver injury. *Stem Cell Res Ther*. (2015) 6:20. doi: 10.1186/s13287-015-0019-z

95. Um S, Kim HY, Lee JH, Song IS, Seo BM. TSG-6 secreted by mesenchymal stem cells suppresses immune reactions influenced by BMP-2 through p38 and MEK mitogen-activated protein kinase pathway. *Cell Tissue Res*. (2017) 368:551–61. doi: 10.1007/s00441-017-2581-4
96. Abels ER, Breakefield XO. Introduction to extracellular vesicles: biogenesis, RNA cargo selection, content, release, and uptake. *Cell Mol Neurobiol*. (2016) 36:301–12. doi: 10.1007/s10571-016-0366-z
97. Jung JW, Kwon M, Choi JC, Shin JW, Park IW, Choi BW, et al. Familial occurrence of pulmonary embolism after intravenous, adipose tissue-derived stem cell therapy. *Yonsei Med J*. (2013) 54:1293–6. doi: 10.3349/ymj.2013.54.5.1293
98. Makela T, Takalo R, Arvola O, Haapanen H, Yannopoulos F, Blanco R, et al. Safety and biodistribution study of bone marrow-derived mesenchymal stromal cells and mononuclear cells and the impact of the administration route in an intact porcine model. *Cytotherapy*. (2015) 17:392–402. doi: 10.1016/j.jcyt.2014.12.004
99. Kalra H, Drummen GP, Mathivanan S. Focus on extracellular vesicles: introducing the next small big thing. *Int J Mol Sci*. (2016) 17:170. doi: 10.3390/ijms17020170
100. Lai RC, Tan SS, Yeo RW, Choo AB, Reiner AT, Su Y, et al. MSC secretes at least 3 EV types each with a unique permutation of membrane lipid, protein and RNA. *J Extracell Vesicles*. (2016) 5:29828. doi: 10.3402/jev.v5.29828
101. Hyvarinen K, Holopainen M, Skirdenko V, Ruhanen H, Lehenkari P, Korhonen M, et al. Mesenchymal stromal cells and their extracellular vesicles enhance the anti-inflammatory phenotype of regulatory macrophages by

downregulating the production of interleukin (IL)-23 and IL-22. *Front Immunol*. (2018) 9:771. doi: 10.3389/fimmu.2018.00771

102. Crain SK, Robinson SR, Thane KE, Davis AM, Meola DM, Barton BA, et al. Extracellular vesicles from Wharton's Jelly mesenchymal stem cells suppress CD4 expressing T cells through transforming growth factor beta and adenosine signaling in a canine model. *Stem Cells Dev*. (2019) 28:212–26. doi: 10.1089/scd.2018.0097
103. Park KS, Svennerholm K, Shelke GV, Bandeira E, Lasser C, Jang SC, et al. Mesenchymal stromal cell-derived nanovesicles ameliorate bacterial outer membrane vesicle-induced sepsis via IL-10. *Stem Cell Res Ther*. (2019) 10:231. doi: 10.1186/s13287-019-1352-4
104. Khatri M, Richardson LA, Meulia T. Mesenchymal stem cell-derived extracellular vesicles attenuate influenza virus-induced acute lung injury in a pig model. *Stem Cell Res Ther*. (2018) 9:17. doi: 10.1186/s13287-018-0774-8
105. Eirin A, Zhu XY, Puranik AS, Tang H, McGurren KA, van Wijnen AJ, et al. Mesenchymal stem cell-derived extracellular vesicles attenuate kidney inflammation. *Kidney Int*. (2017) 92:114–24. doi: 10.1016/j.kint.2016.12.023
106. Haga H, Yan IK, Takahashi K, Matsuda A, Patel T. Extracellular vesicles from bone marrow-derived mesenchymal stem cells improve survival from lethal hepatic failure in mice. *Stem Cells Transl Med*. (2017) 6:1262–72. doi: 10.1002/sctm.16-0226
107. Cosenza S, Ruiz M, Toupet K, Jorgensen C, Noel D. Mesenchymal stem cells derived exosomes and microparticles protect cartilage and bone from degradation in osteoarthritis. *Sci Rep*. (2017) 7:16214. doi: 10.1038/s41598-017-15376-8

108. Ruppert KA, Nguyen TT, Prabhakara KS, Toledano Furman NE, Srivastava AK, Harting MT, et al. Human mesenchymal stromal cell-derived extracellular vesicles modify microglial response and improve clinical outcomes in experimental spinal cord injury. *Sci Rep*. (2018) 8:480. doi: 10.1038/s41598-017-18867-w
109. Deng M, Xiao H, Zhang H, Peng H, Yuan H, Xu Y, et al. Mesenchymal stem cell-derived extracellular vesicles ameliorates hippocampal synaptic impairment after transient global ischemia. *Front Cell Neurosci*. (2017) 11:205. doi: 10.3389/fncel.2017.00205
110. Liu L, Jin X, Hu CF, Li R, Zhou Z, Shen CX. Exosomes derived from mesenchymal stem cells rescue myocardial ischaemia/reperfusion injury by inducing cardiomyocyte autophagy via AMPK and Akt pathways. *Cell Physiol Biochem*. (2017) 43:52–68. doi: 10.1159/000480317
111. Kornicka-Garbowska K, Pedziwiatr R, Wozniak P, Kucharczyk K, Marycz K. Microvesicles isolated from 5-azacytidine-and-resveratrol-treated mesenchymal stem cells for the treatment of suspensory ligament injury in horse-a case report. *Stem Cell Res Ther*. (2019) 10:394. doi: 10.1186/s13287-019-1469-5
112. El-Tookhy OS, Shamaa AA, Shehab GG, Abdallah AN, Azzam OM. Histological evaluation of experimentally induced critical size defect skin wounds using exosomal solution of mesenchymal stem cells derived microvesicles. *Int J Stem Cells*. (2017) 10:144–53. doi: 10.15283/ijsc17043
113. Fu QL, Chow YY, Sun SJ, Zeng QX, Li HB, Shi JB, et al. Mesenchymal stem cells derived from human induced pluripotent stem cells modulate T-cell phenotypes in allergic rhinitis. *Allergy*. (2012) 67:1215–22. doi: 10.1111/j.1398-9995.2012.02875.x

114. Luk F, de Witte SF, Korevaar SS, Roemeling-van Rhijn M, Franquesa M, Strini T, et al. Inactivated mesenchymal stem cells maintain immunomodulatory capacity. *Stem Cells Dev.* (2016) 25:1342–54. doi: 10.1089/scd.2016.0068

115. Tan SS, Yin Y, Lee T, Lai RC, Yeo RW, Zhang B, et al. Therapeutic MSC exosomes are derived from lipid raft microdomains in the plasma membrane. *J Extracell Vesicles.* (2013) 2:22614. doi: 10.3402/jev.v2i0.22614

116. Toh WS, Zhang B, Lai RC, Lim SK. Immune regulatory targets of mesenchymal stromal cell exosomes/small extracellular vesicles in tissue regeneration. *Cytotherapy.* (2018) 20:1419–26. doi: 10.1016/j.jcyt.2018.09.008

117. Reiner AT, Witwer KW, van Balkom BWM, de Beer J, Brodie C, Corteling RL, et al. Concise review: developing best-practice models for the therapeutic use of extracellular vesicles. *Stem Cells Transl Med.* (2017) 6:1730–9. doi: 10.1002/sctm.17-0055

118. Thery C, Witwer KW, Aikawa E, Alcaraz MJ, Anderson JD, Andriantsitohaina R, et al. Minimal information for studies of extracellular vesicles 2018. (MISEV2018): a position statement of the International Society for Extracellular Vesicles and update of the MISEV2014 guidelines. *J Extracell Vesicles.* (2018). 7:1535750. doi: 10.1080/20013078.2018.1461450

119. Elliott MR, Koster KM, Murphy PS. Efferocytosis signaling in the regulation of macrophage inflammatory responses. *J Immunol.* (2017) 198:1387–94. doi: 10.4049/jimmunol.1601520

120. Galleu A, Riffo-Vasquez Y, Trento C, Lomas C, Dolcetti L, Cheung TS, et al. Apoptosis in mesenchymal stromal cells induces *in vivo* recipient-mediated

immunomodulation. *Sci Transl Med*. (2017) 9:eaam7828. doi: 10.1126/scitranslmed.aam7828

121. Cheung TS, Galleu A, von Bonin M, Bornhauser M, Dazzi F. Apoptotic mesenchymal stromal cells induce prostaglandin E2 in monocytes: implications for the monitoring of mesenchymal stromal cell activity. *Haematologica*. (2019) 104:e438–41. doi: 10.3324/haematol.2018.214767
122. de Witte SFH, Luk F, Sierra Parraga JM, Gargesha M, Merino A, Korevaar SS, et al. Immunomodulation by therapeutic mesenchymal stromal cells (MSC) is triggered through phagocytosis of MSC by monocytic cells. *Stem Cells*. (2018) 36:602–15. doi: 10.1002/stem.2779
123. Spees JL, Olson SD, Whitney MJ, Prockop DJ. Mitochondrial transfer between cells can rescue aerobic respiration. *Proc Natl Acad Sci USA*. (2006) 103:1283–8. doi: 10.1073/pnas.0510511103
124. Jackson MV, Morrison TJ, Doherty DF, McAuley DF, Matthay MA, Kissenpfennig A, et al. Mitochondrial transfer via tunneling nanotubes is an important mechanism by which mesenchymal stem cells enhance macrophage phagocytosis in the *in vitro* and *in vivo* models of ARDS. *Stem Cells*. (2016) 34:2210–23. doi: 10.1002/stem.2372
125. Li C, Cheung MKH, Han S, Zhang Z, Chen L, Chen J, et al. Mesenchymal stem cells and their mitochondrial transfer: a double-edged sword. *Biosci Rep*. (2019) 39:BSR20182417. doi: 10.1042/BSR20182417
126. Penn MS. SDF-1:CXCR4 axis is fundamental for tissue preservation and repair. *Am J Pathol*. (2010) 177:2166–8. doi: 10.2353/ajpath.2010.100803
127. Wynn RF, Hart CA, Corradi-Perini C, O'Neill L, Evans CA, Wraith JE, et al. A small proportion of mesenchymal stem cells strongly expresses functionally

active CXCR4 receptor capable of promoting migration to bone marrow. *Blood*. (2004) 104:2643–5. doi: 10.1182/blood-2004-02-0526

128. Chamberlain G, Wright K, Rot A, Ashton B, Middleton J. Murine mesenchymal stem cells exhibit a restricted repertoire of functional chemokine receptors: comparison with human. *PLoS ONE*. (2008) 3:e2934. doi: 10.1371/journal.pone.0002934
129. Zou C, Song G, Luo Q, Yuan L, Yang L. Mesenchymal stem cells require integrin β1 for directed migration induced by osteopontin *in vitro*. *In Vitro Cell Dev Biol Anim*. (2011) 47:241–50. doi: 10.1007/s11626-010-9377-0
130. Wang X, Zhen L, Miao H, Sun Q, Yang Y, Que B, et al. Concomitant retrograde coronary venous infusion of basic fibroblast growth factor enhances engraftment and differentiation of bone marrow mesenchymal stem cells for cardiac repair after myocardial infarction. *Theranostics*. (2015) 5:995–1006. doi: 10.7150/thno.11607
131. Ball SG, Shuttleworth CA, Kielty CM. Vascular endothelial growth factor can signal through platelet-derived growth factor receptors. *J Cell Biol*. (2007) 177:489–500. doi: 10.1083/jcb.200608093
132. Forte G, Minieri M, Cossa P, Antenucci D, Sala M, Gnocchi V, et al. Hepatocyte growth factor effects on mesenchymal stem cells: proliferation, migration, and differentiation. *Stem Cells*. (2006) 24:23–33. doi: 10.1634/stemcells.2004-0176
133. Xinaris C, Morigi M, Benedetti V, Imberti B, Fabricio AS, Squarcina E, et al. A novel strategy to enhance mesenchymal stem cell migration capacity and promote tissue repair in an injury specific fashion. *Cell Transplant*. (2013) 22:423–36. doi: 10.3727/096368912X653246

134. Gao P, Zhou Y, Xian L, Li C, Xu T, Plunkett B, et al. Functional effects of TGF-β1 on mesenchymal stem cell mobilization in cockroach allergen-induced asthma. *J Immunol.* (2014) 192:4560–70. doi: 10.4049/jimmunol.1303461

135. Fu X, Liu G, Halim A, Ju Y, Luo Q, Song AG. Mesenchymal stem cell migration and tissue repair. *Cells.* (2019) 8:784. doi: 10.3390/cells8080784

136. Nowakowski A, Walczak P, Lukomska B, Janowski M. Genetic engineering of mesenchymal stem cells to induce their migration and survival. *Stem Cells Int.* (2016) 2016:4956063. doi: 10.1155/2016/4956063

137. Ullah M, Liu DD, Thakor AS. Mesenchymal stromal cell homing: mechanisms and strategies for improvement. *iScience.* (2019) 15:421–38. doi: 10.1016/j.isci.2019.05.004

138. Gao J, Dennis JE, Muzic RF, Lundberg M, Caplan AI. The dynamic *in vivo* distribution of bone marrow-derived mesenchymal stem cells after infusion. *Cells Tissues Organs.* (2001) 169:12–20. doi: 10.1159/000047856

139. Eggenhofer E, Benseler V, Kroemer A, Popp FC, Geissler EK, Schlitt HJ, et al. Mesenchymal stem cells are short-lived and do not migrate beyond the lungs after intravenous infusion. *Front Immunol.* (2012) 3:297. doi: 10.3389/fimmu.2012.00297

140. Jasmin, Jelicks LA, Tanowitz HB, Peters VM, Mendez-Otero R, de Carvalho ACC, et al. Molecular imaging, biodistribution and efficacy of mesenchymal bone marrow cell therapy in a mouse model of Chagas disease. *Microbes Infect.* (2014) 16:923–35. doi: 10.1016/j.micinf.2014.08.016

141. Kraitchman DL, Tatsumi M, Gilson WD, Ishimori T, Kedziorek D, Walczak P, et al. Dynamic imaging of allogeneic mesenchymal stem cells trafficking to

myocardial infarction. *Circulation*. (2005) 112:1451–61. doi: 10.1161/CIRCULATIONAHA.105.537480

142. Yan Y, Fang J, Wen X, Teng X, Li B, Zhou Z, et al. Therapeutic applications of adipose-derived mesenchymal stem cells on acute liver injury in canines. *Res Vet Sci*. (2019) 126:233–9. doi: 10.1016/j.rvsc.2019.09.004
143. Wang S, Guo L, Ge J, Yu L, Cai T, Tian R, et al. Excess integrins cause lung entrapment of mesenchymal stem cells. *Stem Cells*. (2015) 33:3315–26. doi: 10.1002/stem.2087
144. Abe T, Sumi K, Kunimatsu R, Oki N, Tsuka Y, Awada T, et al. Bone regeneration in a canine model of artificial jaw cleft using bone marrow-derived mesenchymal stem cells and carbonate hydroxyapatite carrier. *Cleft Palate Craniofac J*. (2020) 57:208–17. doi: 10.1177/1055665619868868
145. Sole A, Spriet M, Padgett KA, Vaughan B, Galuppo LD, Borjesson DL, et al. Distribution and persistence of technetium-99 hexamethyl propylene amine oxime-labelled bone marrow-derived mesenchymal stem cells in experimentally induced tendon lesions after intratendinous injection and regional perfusion of the equine distal limb. *Equine Vet J*. (2013) 45:726–31. doi: 10.1111/evj.12063
146. Walczak P, Zhang J, Gilad AA, Kedziorek DA, Ruiz-Cabello J, Young RG, et al. Dual-modality monitoring of targeted intraarterial delivery of mesenchymal stem cells after transient ischemia. *Stroke*. (2008) 39:1569–74. doi: 10.1161/STROKEAHA.107.502047
147. Trela JM, Spriet M, Padgett KA, Galuppo LD, Vaughan B, Vidal MA. Scintigraphic comparison of intra-arterial injection and distal intravenous regional limb perfusion for administration of mesenchymal stem cells to the equine foot. *Equine Vet J*. (2014) 46:479–83. doi: 10.1111/evj.12137

148. Torrent A, Spriet M, Espinosa-Mur P, Clark KC, Whitcomb MB, Borjesson DL, et al. Ultrasound-guided injection of the cranial tibial artery for stem cell administration in horses. *Equine Vet J.* (2019) 51:681–7. doi: 10.1111/evj.13065
149. Nishimura T, Takami T, Sasaki R, Aibe Y, Matsuda T, Fujisawa K, et al. Liver regeneration therapy through the hepatic artery-infusion of cultured bone marrow cells in a canine liver fibrosis model. *PLoS ONE.* (2019) 14:e0210588. doi: 10.1371/journal.pone.0210588
150. Parys M, Nelson N, Koehl K, Miller R, Kaneene JB, Kruger JM, et al. Safety of intraperitoneal injection of adipose tissue-derived autologous mesenchymal stem cells in cats. *J Vet Intern Med.* (2016) 30:157–63. doi: 10.1111/jvim.13655
151. Wiafe B, Kadam R, Metcalfe PD. Intraperitoneal administration of mesenchymal stem cells is effective at mitigating detrusor deterioration after pBOO. *Am J Physiol Renal Physiol.* (2020) 318:F549–56. doi: 10.1152/ajprenal.00486.2019
152. Gooch A, Zhang P, Hu Z, Loy Son N, Avila N, Fischer J, et al. Interim report on the effective intraperitoneal therapy of insulin-dependent diabetes mellitus in pet dogs using "Neo-Islets," aggregates of adipose stem and pancreatic islet cells (INAD 012-776). *PLoS ONE.* (2019) 14:e0218688. doi: 10.1371/journal.pone.0218688
153. Le Blanc K, Tammik C, Rosendahl K, Zetterberg E, Ringdén O. HLA expression and immunologic propertiesof differentiated and undifferentiated mesenchymal stem cells. *Exp Hematol.* (2003) 31:890–6. doi: 10.1016/S0301-472X(03)00110-3

154. Klyushnenkova E, Mosca JD, Zernetkina V, Majumdar MK, Beggs KJ, Simonetti DW, et al. T cell responses to allogeneic human mesenchymal stem cells: immunogenicity, tolerance, and suppression. *J Biomed Sci.* (2005) 12:47–57. doi: 10.1007/s11373-004-8183-7
155. van Megen KM, van 't Wout ET, Lages Motta J, Dekker B, Nikolic T, Roep BO. Activated mesenchymal stromal cells process and present antigens regulating adaptive immunity. *Front Immunol.* (2019) 10:694. doi: 10.3389/fimmu.2019.00694
156. Sivanathan KN, Rojas-Canales D, Grey ST, Gronthos S, Coates PT. Transcriptome profiling of IL-17A preactivated mesenchymal stem cells: a comparative study to unmodified and IFN-γ modified mesenchymal stem cells. *Stem Cells Int.* (2017) 2017:1025820. doi: 10.1155/2017/1025820
157. Li X, Shang B, Li YN, Shi Y, Shao C. IFNγ and TNFα synergistically induce apoptosis of mesenchymal stem/stromal cells via the induction of nitric oxide. *Stem Cell Res Ther.* (2019) 10:18. doi: 10.1186/s13287-018-1102-z
158. Brandt L, Schubert S, Scheibe P, Brehm W, Franzen J, Gross C, et al. Tenogenic properties of mesenchymal progenitor cells are compromised in an inflammatory environment. *Int J Mol Sci.* (2018) 19:2549. doi: 10.3390/ijms19092549
159. Dakin SG, Jespers K, Warner S, O'Hara LK, Dudhia J, Goodship AE, et al. The relationship between *in vivo* limb and *in vitro* tendon mechanics after injury: a potential novel clinical tool for monitoring tendon repair. *Equine Vet J.* (2011) 43:418–23. doi: 10.1111/j.2042-3306.2010.00303.x
160. Dyson SJ. Medical management of superficial digital flexor tendonitis: a comparative study in 219 horses (1992-2000). *Equine Vet J.* (2004) 36:415–9. doi: 10.2746/0425164044868422

161. Petrov R, MacDonald MH, Tesch AM, Van Hoogmoed LM. Influence of topically applied cold treatment on core temperature and cell viability in equine superficial digital flexor tendons. *Am J Vet Res*. (2003) 64:835–44. doi: 10.2460/ajvr.2003.64.835
162. Chan KM, Fu SC. Anti-inflammatory management for tendon injuries - friends or foes? *Sports Med Arthrosc Rehabil Ther Technol*. (2009) 1:23. doi: 10.1186/1758-2555-1-23
163. Jann HW, Stein LE, Good JK. Strength characteristics and failure modes of locking-loop and three-loop pulley suture patterns in equine tendons. *Vet Surg*. (1990) 19:28–33. doi: 10.1111/j.1532-950X.1990.tb01139.x
164. Eliashar E, Schramme MC, Schumacher J, Ikada Y, Smith RK. Use of a bioabsorbable implant for the repair of severed digital flexor tendons in four horses. *Vet Rec*. (2001) 148:506–9. doi: 10.1136/vr.148.16.506
165. Smith RK, Korda M, Blunn GW, Goodship AE. Isolation and implantation of autologous equine mesenchymal stem cells from bone marrow into the superficial digital flexor tendon as a potential novel treatment. *Equine Vet J*. (2003) 35:99–102. doi: 10.2746/042516403775467388
166. Renzi S, Ricco S, Dotti S, Sesso L, Grolli S, Cornali M, et al. Autologous bone marrow mesenchymal stromal cells for regeneration of injured equine ligaments and tendons: a clinical report. *Res Vet Sci*. (2013) 95:272–7. doi: 10.1016/j.rvsc.2013.01.017
167. Filomeno P, Dayan V, Tourino C. Stem cell research and clinical development in tendon repair. *Muscles Ligaments Tendons J*. (2012) 2:204–11.

168. Costa-Almeida R, Calejo I, Gomes ME. Mesenchymal stem cells empowering tendon regenerative therapies. *Int J Mol Sci*. (2019) 20:3002. doi: 10.3390/ijms20123002
169. Pacini S, Spinabella S, Trombi L, Fazzi R, Galimberti S, Dini F, et al. Suspension of bone marrow-derived undifferentiated mesenchymal stromal cells for repair of superficial digital flexor tendon in race horses. *Tissue Eng*. (2007) 13:2949–55. doi: 10.1089/ten.2007.0108
170. Godwin EE, Young NJ, Dudhia J, Beamish IC, Smith RK. Implantation of bone marrow-derived mesenchymal stem cells demonstrates improved outcome in horses with overstrain injury of the superficial digital flexor tendon. *Equine Vet J*. (2012) 44:25–32. doi: 10.1111/j.2042-3306.2011.00363.x
171. Smith RK, Werling NJ, Dakin SG, Alam R, Goodship AE, Dudhia J. Beneficial effects of autologous bone marrow-derived mesenchymal stem cells in naturally occurring tendinopathy. *PLoS ONE*. (2013) 8:e75697. doi: 10.1371/journal.pone.0075697
172. Van Loon VJ, Scheffer CJ, Genn HJ, Hoogendoorn AC, Greve JW. Clinical follow-up of horses treated with allogeneic equine mesenchymal stem cells derived from umbilical cord blood for different tendon and ligament disorders. *Vet Q*. (2014) 34:92–7. doi: 10.1080/01652176.2014.949390
173. Geburek F, Roggel F, van Schie HTM, Beineke A, Estrada R, Weber K, et al. Effect of single intralesional treatment of surgically induced equine superficial digital flexor tendon core lesions with adipose-derived mesenchymal stromal cells: a controlled experimental trial. *Stem Cell Res Ther*. (2017) 8:129. doi: 10.1186/s13287-017-0564-8

174. Romero A, Barrachina L, Ranera B, Remacha AR, Moreno B, de Blas I, et al. Comparison of autologous bone marrow and adipose tissue derived mesenchymal stem cells, and platelet rich plasma, for treating surgically induced lesions of the equine superficial digital flexor tendon. *Vet J.* (2017) 224:76–84. doi: 10.1016/j.tvjl.2017.04.005
175. Harasen G. Diagnosing rupture of the cranial cruciate ligament. *Can Vet J.* (2002) 43:475–6.
176. Chuang C, Ramaker MA, Kaur S, Csomos RA, Kroner KT, Bleedorn JA, et al. Radiographic risk factors for contralateral rupture in dogs with unilateral cranial cruciate ligament rupture. *PLoS ONE.* (2014) 9:e106389. doi: 10.1371/journal.pone.0106389
177. Molsa SH, Hyytiainen HK, Hielm-Bjorkman AK, Laitinen-Vapaavuori OM. Long-term functional outcome after surgical repair of cranial cruciate ligament disease in dogs. *BMC Vet Res.* (2014) 10:266. doi: 10.1186/s12917-014-0266-8
178. Taroni M, Cabon Q, Febre M, Cachon T, Saulnier N, Carozzo C, et al. Evaluation of the effect of a single intra-articular injection of allogeneic neonatal mesenchymal stromal cells compared to oral non-steroidal anti-inflammatory treatment on the postoperative musculoskeletal status and gait of dogs over a 6-month period after tibial plateau leveling osteotomy: a pilot study. *Front Vet Sci.* (2017) 4:83. doi: 10.3389/fvets.2017.00083
179. Linon E, Spreng D, Rytz U, Forterre S. Engraftment of autologous bone marrow cells into the injured cranial cruciate ligament in dogs. *Vet J.* (2014) 202:448–54. doi: 10.1016/j.tvjl.2014.08.031
180. Muir P, Hans EC, Racette M, Volstad N, Sample SJ, Heaton C, et al. Autologous bone marrow-derived mesenchymal stem cells modulate

molecular markers of inflammation in dogs with cruciate ligament rupture. *PLoS ONE*. (2016) 11:e0159095. doi: 10.1371/journal.pone.0159095

181. Canapp SO Jr, Leasure CS, Cox C, Ibrahim V, Carr BJ. Partial cranial cruciate ligament tears treated with stem cell and platelet-rich plasma combination therapy in 36 dogs: a retrospective study. *Front Vet Sci*. (2016) 3:112. doi: 10.3389/fvets.2016.00112
182. Frisbie DD, Stewart MC. Cell-based therapies for equine joint disease. *Vet Clin North Am Equine Pract*. (2011) 27:335–49. doi: 10.1016/j.cveq.2011.06.005
183. Rossdale PD, Hopes R, Digby NJ, offord K. Epidemiological study of wastage among racehorses 1982 and (1983). *Vet Rec*. (1985) 116:66–9. doi: 10.1136/vr.116.3.66
184. Walmsley JR, Phillips TJ, Townsend HG. Meniscal tears in horses: an evaluation of clinical signs and arthroscopic treatment of 80 cases. *Equine Vet J*. (2003) 35:402–6. doi: 10.2746/042516403776014163
185. Cohen JM, Richardson DW, McKnight AL, Ross MW, Boston RC. Long-term outcome in 44 horses with stifle lameness after arthroscopic exploration and debridement. *Vet Surg*. (2009) 38:543–51. doi: 10.1111/j.1532-950X.2009.00524.x
186. Nicpon J, Marycz K, Grzesiak J. Therapeutic effect of adipose-derived mesenchymal stem cell injection in horses suffering from bone spavin. *Pol J Vet Sci*. (2013) 16:753–4. doi: 10.2478/pjvs-2013-0107
187. Ferris DJ, Frisbie DD, Kisiday JD, McIlwraith CW, Hague BA, Major MD, et al. Clinical outcome after intra-articular administration of bone marrow derived mesenchymal stem cells in 33 horses with stifle injury. *Vet Surg*. (2014) 43:255–65. doi: 10.1111/j.1532-950X.2014.12100.x

188. Marinas-Pardo L, Garcia-Castro J, Rodriguez-Hurtado I, Rodriguez-Garcia MI, Nunez-Naveira L, Hermida-Prieto M. Allogeneic adipose-derived mesenchymal stem cells (horse allo 20) for the treatment of osteoarthritis-associated lameness in horses: characterization, safety, and efficacy of intra-articular treatment. *Stem Cells Dev.* (2018) 27:1147–60. doi: 10.1089/scd.2018.0074
189. Mohoric L, Zorko B, Ceh K, Majdic G. Blinded placebo study of bilateral osteoarthritis treatment using adipose derived mesenchymal stem cells. *Slovenian Vet Res.* (2016) 53:167–74.
190. Black LL, Gaynor J, Gahring D, Adams C, Aron D, Harman S, et al. Effect of adipose-derived mesenchymal stem and regenerative cells on lameness in dogs with chronic osteoarthritis of the coxofemoral joints: a randomized, double-blinded, multicenter, controlled trial. *Vet Ther.* (2007) 8:272–84.
191. Vilar JM, Morales M, Santana A, Spinella G, Rubio M, Cuervo B, et al. Controlled, blinded force platform analysis of the effect of intraarticular injection of autologous adipose-derived mesenchymal stem cells associated to PRGF-Endoret in osteoarthritic dogs. *BMC Vet Res.* (2013) 9:131. doi: 10.1186/1746-6148-9-131
192. Srzentic Drazilov S, Mrkovacki J, Spasovski V, Fazlagic A, Pavlovic S, Nikcevic G. The use of canine mesenchymal stem cells for the autologous treatment of osteoarthritis. *Acta Vet Hung.* (2018) 66:376–89. doi: 10.1556/004.2018.034
193. Harman R, Carlson K, Gaynor J, Gustafson S, Dhupa S, Clement K, et al. A prospective, randomized, masked, and placebo-controlled efficacy study of intraarticular allogeneic adipose stem cells for the treatment of osteoarthritis in dogs. *Front Vet Sci.* (2016) 3:81. doi: 10.3389/fvets.2016.00081

194. Shah K, Drury T, Roic I, Hansen P, Malin M, Boyd R, et al. Outcome of allogeneic adult stem cell therapy in dogs suffering from osteoarthritis and other joint defects. *Stem Cells Int.* (2018) 2018:7309201. doi: 10.1155/2018/7309201
195. Li L, Duan X, Fan Z, Chen L, Xing F, Xu Z, et al. Mesenchymal stem cells in combination with hyaluronic acid for articular cartilage defects. *Sci Rep.* (2018) 8:9900. doi: 10.1038/s41598-018-27737-y
196. Guercio A, Di Marco P, Casella S, Cannella V, Russotto L, Purpari G, et al. Production of canine mesenchymal stem cells from adipose tissue and their application in dogs with chronic osteoarthritis of the humeroradial joints. *Cell Biol Int.* (2012) 36:189–94. doi: 10.1042/CBI20110304
197. Cuervo B, Rubio M, Sopena J, Dominguez JM, Vilar J, Morales M, et al. Hip osteoarthritis in dogs: a randomized study using mesenchymal stem cells from adipose tissue and plasma rich in growth factors. *Int J Mol Sci.* (2014) 15:13437–60. doi: 10.3390/ijms150813437
198. Babu NC, Gomes AJ. Systemic manifestations of oral diseases. *J Oral Maxillofac Pathol.* (2011) 15:144–7. doi: 10.4103/0973-029X.84477
199. Petersen PE, Bourgeois D, Ogawa H, Estupinan-Day S, Ndiaye C. The global burden of oral diseases and risks to oral health. *Bull World Health Organ.* (2005) 83:661–9.
200. Abdelaz P, ElZoghbi A, Shokry M, Ahmed AZ, Rasha H. Reparative dentin formation using stem cell therapy versus calcium hydroxide in direct pulp capping: an animal study. *Braz Dent J.* (2019) 30:542–9. doi: 10.1590/0103-6440201902711
201. Iohara K, Utsunomiya S, Kohara S, Nakashima M. Allogeneic transplantation of mobilized dental pulp stem cells with the mismatched dog leukocyte

antigen type is safe and efficacious for total pulp regeneration. *Stem Cell Res Ther*. (2018) 9:116. doi: 10.1186/s13287-018-0855-8

202. Colpak HA, Gonen ZB, Ozdamar S, Alkan A, Kutuk N. Vertical ridge augmentation using guided bone regeneration procedure and dental pulp derived mesenchymal stem cells with simultaneous dental implant placement: a histologic study in a sheep model. *J Stomatol Oral Maxillofac Surg*. (2019) 120:216–23. doi: 10.1016/j.jormas.2018.12.011
203. Shi H, Zong W, Xu X, Chen J. Improved biphasic calcium phosphate combined with periodontal ligament stem cells may serve as a promising method for periodontal regeneration. *Am J Transl Res*. (2018) 10:4030–41.
204. Wang P, Wang W, Geng T, Liu Y, Zhu S, Liu Z, et al. EphrinB2 regulates osteogenic differentiation of periodontal ligament stem cells and alveolar bone defect regeneration in beagles. *J Tissue Eng*. (2019) 10:2041731419894361. doi: 10.1177/2041731419894361
205. Xu M, Wei X, Fang J, Xiao L. Combination of SDF-1 and bFGF promotes bone marrow stem cell-mediated periodontal ligament regeneration. *Biosci Rep*. (2019) 39:BSR20190785. doi: 10.1042/BSR20190785
206. Rezaei M, Jamshidi S, Saffarpour A, Ashouri M, Rahbarghazi R, Rokn AR, et al. Transplantation of bone marrow-derived mesenchymal stem cells, platelet-rich plasma, and fibrin glue for periodontal regeneration. *Int J Periodont Restor Dent*. (2019) 39:e32–45. doi: 10.11607/prd.3691
207. Venkataiah VS, Handa K, Njuguna MM, Hasegawa T, Maruyama K, Nemoto E, et al. Periodontal regeneration by allogeneic transplantation of adipose tissue derived multi-lineage progenitor stem cells *in vivo*. *Sci Rep*. (2019) 9:921. doi: 10.1038/s41598-018-37528-0

208. El-Zekrid MH, Mahmoud SH, Ali FA, Helal ME, Grawish ME. Healing capacity of autologous bone marrow-derived mesenchymal stem cells on partially pulpotomized dogs' teeth. *J Endod*. (2019) 45:287–94. doi: 10.1016/j.joen.2018.11.013

209. Sanchez-Garces MA, Alvira-Gonzalez J, Sanchez CM, Barbany Cairo JR, Del Pozo MR, Gay-Escoda C. Bone regeneration using adipose-derived stem cells with fibronectin in dehiscence-type defects associated with dental implants: an experimental study in a dog model. *Int J Oral Maxillofac Implants*. (2017) 32:e97–e106. doi: 10.11607/jomi.5169

210. Bellei E, Dalla F, Masetti L, Pisoni L, Joechler M. Surgical therapy in chronic feline gingivostomatitis (FCGS). *Vet Res Commun*. (2008) 32(Suppl. 1):S231–4. doi: 10.1007/s11259-008-9153-8

211. Hennet PR, Camy GA, McGahie DM, Albouy MV. Comparative efficacy of a recombinant feline interferon omega in refractory cases of calicivirus-positive cats with caudal stomatitis: a randomised, multi-centre, controlled, double-blind study in 39 cats. *J Feline Med Surg*. (2011) 13:577–87. doi: 10.1016/j.jfms.2011.05.012

212. Lommer MJ. Efficacy of cyclosporine for chronic, refractory stomatitis in cats: a randomized, placebo-controlled, double-blinded clinical study. *J Vet Dent*. (2013) 30:8–17. doi: 10.1177/089875641303000101

213. Druet I, Hennet P. Relationship between feline calicivirus load, oral lesions, and outcome in feline chronic gingivostomatitis (caudal stomatitis): retrospective study in 104 cats. *Front Vet Sci*. (2017) 4:209. doi: 10.3389/fvets.2017.00209

214. Winer JN, Arzi B, Verstraete FJ. Therapeutic management of feline chronic gingivostomatitis: a systematic review of the literature. *Front Vet Sci.* (2016) 3:54. doi: 10.3389/fvets.2016.00054
215. Arzi B, Mills-Ko E, Verstraete FJ, Kol A, Walker NJ, Badgley MR, et al. Therapeutic efficacy of fresh, autologous mesenchymal stem cells for severe refractory gingivostomatitis in cats. *Stem Cells Transl Med.* (2016) 5:75–86. doi: 10.5966/sctm.2015-0127
216. Arzi B, Clark KC, Sundaram A, Spriet M, Verstraete FJM, Walker NJ, et al. Therapeutic efficacy of fresh, allogeneic mesenchymal stem cells for severe refractory feline chronic gingivostomatitis. *Stem Cells Transl Med.* (2017) 6:1710–22. doi: 10.1002/sctm.17-0035
217. Arzi B, Peralta S, Fiani N, Vapniarsky N, Taechangam N, Delatorre U, et al. A multicenter experience using adipose-derived mesenchymal stem cell therapy for cats with chronic, non-responsive gingivostomatitis. *Stem Cell Res Ther.* (2020) 11:115. doi: 10.1186/s13287-020-01623-9
218. Cerquetella M, Spaterna A, Laus F, Tesei B, Rossi G, Antonelli E, et al. Inflammatory bowel disease in the dog: differences and similarities with humans. *World J Gastroenterol.* (2010) 16:1050–6. doi: 10.3748/wjg.v16.i9.1050
219. Perez-Merino EM, Uson-Casaus JM, Duque-Carrasco J, Zaragoza-Bayle C, Marinas-Pardo L, Hermida-Prieto M, et al. Safety and efficacy of allogeneic adipose tissue-derived mesenchymal stem cells for treatment of dogs with inflammatory bowel disease: Endoscopic and histological outcomes. *Vet J.* (2015) 206:391–7. doi: 10.1016/j.tvjl.2015.07.023

220. Webb TL, Webb CB. Stem cell therapy in cats with chronic enteropathy: a proof-of-concept study. *J Feline Med Surg*. (2015) 17:901–8. doi: 10.1177/1098612X14561105

221. Matsuda T, Takami T, Sasaki R, Nishimura T, Aibe Y, Paredes BD, et al. A canine liver fibrosis model to develop a therapy for liver cirrhosis using cultured bone marrow-derived cells. *Hepatol Commun*. (2017) 1:691–703. doi: 10.1002/hep4.1071

222. Gardin C, Ferroni L, Bellin G, Rubini G, Barosio S, Zavan B. Therapeutic potential of autologous adipose-derived stem cells for the treatment of liver disease. *Int J Mol Sci*. (2018) 19:4064. doi: 10.3390/ijms19124064

223. Nam A, Han SM, Go DM, Kim DY, Seo KW, Youn HY. Long-term management with adipose tissue-derived mesenchymal stem cells and conventional treatment in a dog with hepatocutaneous syndrome. *J Vet Intern Med*. (2017) 31:1514–9. doi: 10.1111/jvim.14798

224. Adin CA, Gregory CR, Kyles AE, Cowgill L. Diagnostic predictors of complications and survival after renal transplantation in cats. *Vet Surg*. (2001) 30:515–21. doi: 10.1053/jvet.2001.28418

225. Quimby JM, Webb TL, Gibbons DS, Dow SW. Evaluation of intrarenal mesenchymal stem cell injection for treatment of chronic kidney disease in cats: a pilot study. *J Feline Med Surg*. (2011) 13:418–26. doi: 10.1016/j.jfms.2011.01.005

226. Vidane AS, Pinheiro AO, Casals JB, Passarelli D, Hage M, Bueno RS, et al. Transplantation of amniotic membrane-derived multipotent cells ameliorates and delays the progression of chronic kidney disease in cats. *Reprod Domest Anim*. (2017) 52(Suppl. 2):316–26. doi: 10.1111/rda.12846

227. Quimby JM, Webb TL, Habenicht LM, Dow SW. Safety and efficacy of intravenous infusion of allogeneic cryopreserved mesenchymal stem cells for treatment of chronic kidney disease in cats: results of three sequential pilot studies. *Stem Cell Res Ther*. (2013) 4:48. doi: 10.1186/scrt198
228. Quimby JM, Webb TL, Randall E, Marolf A, Valdes-Martinez A, Dow SW. Assessment of intravenous adipose-derived allogeneic mesenchymal stem cells for the treatment of feline chronic kidney disease: a randomized, placebo-controlled clinical trial in eight cats. *J Feline Med Surg*. (2016) 18:165–71. doi: 10.1177/1098612X15576980
229. Wernly B, Mirna M, Rezar R, Prodinger C, Jung C, Podesser BK, et al. Regenerative cardiovascular therapies: stem cells and beyond. *Int J Mol Sci*. (2019) 20:1420. doi: 10.3390/ijms20061420
230. Hoffman AM, Dow SW. Concise review: stem cell trials using companion animal disease models. *Stem Cells*. (2016) 34:1709–29. doi: 10.1002/stem.2377
231. Pogue B, Estrada AH, Sosa-Samper I, Maisenbacher HW, Lamb KE, Mincey BD, et al. Stem-cell therapy for dilated cardiomyopathy: a pilot study evaluating retrograde coronary venous delivery. *J Small Anim Pract*. (2013) 54:361–6. doi: 10.1111/jsap.12098
232. Hensley MT, Tang J, Woodruff K, Defrancesco T, Tou S, Williams CM, et al. Intracoronary allogeneic cardiosphere-derived stem cells are safe for use in dogs with dilated cardiomyopathy. *J Cell Mol Med*. (2017) 21:1503–12. doi: 10.1111/jcmm.13077
233. Fox PR. Pathology of myxomatous mitral valve disease in the dog. *J Vet Cardiol*. (2012) 14:103–26. doi: 10.1016/j.jvc.2012.02.001

234. Petchdee S, Sompeewong S. Intravenous administration of puppy deciduous teeth stem cells in degenerative valve disease. *Vet World*. (2016) 9:1429–34. doi: 10.14202/vetworld.2016.1429-1434

235. Barussi FC, Bastos FZ, Leite LM, Fragoso FY, Senegaglia AC, Brofman PR, et al. Intratracheal therapy with autologous bone marrow-derived mononuclear cells reduces airway inflammation in horses with recurrent airway obstruction. *Respir Physiol Neurobiol*. (2016) 232:35–42. doi: 10.1016/j.resp.2016.07.002

236. Hao Y, Ran Y, Lu B, Li J, Zhang J, Feng C, et al. Therapeutic effects of human umbilical cord-derived mesenchymal stem cells on canine radiation-induced lung injury. *Int J Radiat Oncol Biol Phys*. (2018) 102:407–16. doi: 10.1016/j.ijrobp.2018.05.068

237. Trzil JE, Masseau I, Webb TL, Chang CH, Dodam JR, Liu H, et al. Intravenous adipose-derived mesenchymal stem cell therapy for the treatment of feline asthma: a pilot study. *J Feline Med Surg*. (2016) 18:981–90. doi: 10.1177/1098612X15604351

238. Besalti O, Aktas Z, Can P, Akpinar E, Elcin AE, Elcin YM. The use of autologous neurogenically-induced bone marrow-derived mesenchymal stem cells for the treatment of paraplegic dogs without nociception due to spinal trauma. *J Vet Med Sci*. (2016) 78:1465–73. doi: 10.1292/jvms.15-0571

239. Penha EM, Meira CS, Guimaraes ET, Mendonca MV, Gravely FA, Pinheiro CM, et al. Use of autologous mesenchymal stem cells derived from bone marrow for the treatment of naturally injured spinal cord in dogs. *Stem Cells Int*. (2014) 2014:437521. doi: 10.1155/2014/437521

240. Bhat IA, T BS, Somal A, Pandey S, Bharti MK, Panda BSK, et al. An allogenic therapeutic strategy for canine spinal cord injury using

mesenchymal stem cells. *J Cell Physiol*. (2019) 234:2705–18. doi: 10.1002/jcp.27086

241. Bach FS, Rebelatto CLK, Fracaro L, Senegaglia AC, Fragoso FYI, Daga DR, et al. Comparison of the efficacy of surgical decompression alone and combined with canine adipose tissue-derived stem cell transplantation in dogs with acute thoracolumbar disk disease and spinal cord injury. *Front Vet Sci*. (2019) 6:383. doi: 10.3389/fvets.2019.00383
242. Steffen F, Smolders LA, Roentgen AM, Bertolo A, Stoyanov J. Bone marrow-derived mesenchymal stem cells as autologous therapy in dogs with naturally occurring intervertebral disc disease: feasibility, safety, and preliminary results. *Tissue Eng Part C Methods*. (2017) 23:643–51. doi: 10.1089/ten.tec.2017.0033
243. Wu GH, Shi HJ, Che MT, Huang MY, Wei QS, Feng B, et al. Recovery of paralyzed limb motor function in canine with complete spinal cord injury following implantation of MSC-derived neural network tissue. *Biomaterials*. (2018) 181:15–34. doi: 10.1016/j.biomaterials.2018.07.010
244. Ojeh N, Pastar I, Tomic-Canic M, Stojadinovic O. Stem cells in skin regeneration, wound healing, and their clinical applications. *Int J Mol Sci*. (2015) 16:25476–501. doi: 10.3390/ijms161025476
245. Pratheesh MD, Dubey PK, Gade NE, Nath A, Sivanarayanan TB, Madhu DN, et al. Comparative study on characterization and wound healing potential of goat (*Capra hircus*) mesenchymal stem cells derived from fetal origin amniotic fluid and adult bone marrow. *Res Vet Sci*. (2017) 112:81–8. doi: 10.1016/j.rvsc.2016.12.009
246. Martinello T, Gomiero C, Perazzi A, Iacopetti I, Gemignani F, DeBenedictis GM, et al. Allogeneic mesenchymal stem cells improve the wound healing

process of sheep skin. *BMC Vet Res*. (2018) 14:202. doi: 10.1186/s12917-018-1527-8

247. Textor JA, Clark KC, Walker NJ, Aristizobal FA, Kol A, LeJeune SS, et al. Allogeneic stem cells alter gene expression and improve healing of distal limb wounds in horses. *Stem Cells Transl Med*. (2018) 7:98–108. doi: 10.1002/sctm.17-0071
248. Johnson V, Webb T, Norman A, Coy J, Kurihara J, Regan D, et al. Activated mesenchymal stem cells interact with antibiotics and host innate immune responses to control chronic bacterial infections. *Sci Rep*. (2017) 7:9575. doi: 10.1038/s41598-017-08311-4
249. Lanci A, Merlo B, Mariella J, Castagnetti C, Iacono E. Heterologous Wharton's Jelly derived mesenchymal stem cells application on a large chronic skin wound in a 6-month-old filly. *Front Vet Sci*. (2019) 6:9. doi: 10.3389/fvets.2019.00009
250. Hall MN, Rosenkrantz WS, Hong JH, Griffin CE, Mendelsohn CM. Evaluation of the potential use of adipose-derived mesenchymal stromal cells in the treatment of canine atopic dermatitis: a pilot study. *Vet Ther*. (2010) 11:E1–14.
251. Villatoro AJ, Hermida-Prieto M, Fernandez V, Farinas F, Alcoholado C, Rodriguez-Garcia MI, et al. Allogeneic adipose-derived mesenchymal stem cell therapy in dogs with refractory atopic dermatitis: clinical efficacy and safety. *Vet Rec*. (2018) 183:654. doi: 10.1136/vr.104867
252. Davis AB, Schnabel LV, Gilger BC. Subconjunctival bone marrow-derived mesenchymal stem cell therapy as a novel treatment alternative for equine immune-mediated keratitis: a case series. *Vet Ophthalmol*. (2019) 22:674–82. doi: 10.1111/vop.12641

253. Saldinger LK, Nelson SG, Bellone RR, Lassaline M, Mack M, Walker NJ, et al. Horses with equine recurrent uveitis have an activated CD4+ T-cell phenotype that can be modulated by mesenchymal stem cells *in vitro*. *Vet Ophthalmol*. (2020) 23:160–70. doi: 10.1111/vop.12704

254. Villatoro AJ, Claros S, Fernandez V, Alcoholado C, Farinas F, Moreno A, et al. Safety and efficacy of the mesenchymal stem cell in feline eosinophilic keratitis treatment. *BMC Vet Res*. (2018) 14:116. doi: 10.1186/s12917-018-1413-4

255. Villatoro AJ, Fernandez V, Claros S, Rico-Llanos GA, Becerra J, Andrades JA. Use of adipose-derived mesenchymal stem cells in keratoconjunctivitis sicca in a canine model. *Biomed Res Int*. (2015) 2015:527926. doi: 10.1155/2015/527926

256. Sgrignoli MR, Silva DA, Nascimento FF, Sgrignoli DAM, Nai GA, da Silva MG, et al. Reduction in the inflammatory markers CD4, IL-1, IL-6 and TNFα in dogs with keratoconjunctivitis sicca treated topically with mesenchymal stem cells. *Stem Cell Res*. (2019) 39:101525. doi: 10.1016/j.scr.2019.101525

257. Grady ST, Watts AE, Thompson JA, Penedo MCT, Konganti K, Hinrichs K. Effect of intra-ovarian injection of mesenchymal stem cells in aged mares. *J Assist Reprod Genet*. (2019) 36:543–56. doi: 10.1007/s10815-018-1371-6

258. Papa PM, Guasti PN, De Vita B, Nakazato NG, Maia L, Freitas Dell'Aqua CP, et al. Clinical safety of intratesticular transplantation of allogeneic bone marrow multipotent stromal cells in stallions. *Reprod Domest Anim*. (2020) 55:429–37. doi: 10.1111/rda.13624

259. Qamar AY, Fang X, Kim MJ, Cho J. Improved post-thaw quality of canine semen after treatment with exosomes from conditioned medium of adipose-

derived mesenchymal stem cells. *Animals*. (2019) 9:865. doi: 10.3390/ani9110865

260. Lara E, Rivera N, Cabezas J, Navarrete F, Saravia F, Rodriguez-Alvarez L, et al. Endometrial stem cells in farm animals: potential role in uterine physiology and pathology. *Bioengineering*. (2018) 5:75. doi: 10.3390/bioengineering5030075
261. Miernik K, Karasinski J. Porcine uterus contains a population of mesenchymal stem cells. *Reproduction*. (2012) 143:203–9. doi: 10.1530/REP-11-0202
262. Cabezas J, Lara E, Pacha P, Rojas D, Veraguas D, Saravia F, et al. The endometrium of cycling cows contains populations of putative mesenchymal progenitor cells. *Reprod Domest Anim*. (2014) 49:550–9. doi: 10.1111/rda.12309
263. Letouzey V, Tan KS, Deane JA, Ulrich D, Gurung S, Ong YR, et al. Isolation and characterisation of mesenchymal stem/stromal cells in the ovine endometrium. *PLoS ONE*. (2015) 10:e0127531. doi: 10.1371/journal.pone.0127531
264. Tamadon A, Mehrabani D, Zarezadeh Y, Rahmanifar F, Dianatpour M, Zare S. Caprine endometrial mesenchymal stromal stem cell: multilineage potential, characterization, and growth kinetics in breeding and anestrous stages. *Vet Med Int*. (2017) 2017:5052801. doi: 10.1155/2017/5052801
265. Cabezas J, Rojas D, Navarrete F, Ortiz R, Rivera G, Saravia F, et al. Equine mesenchymal stem cells derived from endometrial or adipose tissue share significant biological properties, but have distinctive pattern of surface markers and migration. *Theriogenology*. (2018) 106:93–102. doi: 10.1016/j.theriogenology.2017.09.035

266. Mambelli LI, Winter GH, Kerkis A, Malschitzky E, Mattos RC, Kerkis I. A novel strategy of mesenchymal stem cells delivery in the uterus of mares with endometrosis. *Theriogenology.* (2013) 79:744–50. doi: 10.1016/j.theriogenology.2012.11.030
267. Cahuascanco B, Bahamonde J, Huaman O, Jervis M, Cortez J, Palomino J, et al. Bovine fetal mesenchymal stem cells exert antiproliferative effect against mastitis causing pathogen *Staphylococcus aureus*. *Vet Res*. (2019) 50:25. doi: 10.1186/s13567-019-0643-1
268. 268. Costa CRM, Feitosa MLT, Rocha AR, Bezerra DO, Leite YKC, Argolo Neto NM, et al. Adipose stem cells in reparative goat mastitis mammary gland. *PLoS ONE*. (2019) 14:e0223751. doi: 10.1371/journal.pone.0223751
269. 269. EMA. *Questions and Answers on Allogeneic Stem Cell-Based Products for Veterinary Use: Specific Questions on Extraneous Agents.* (2019). Available online at: https://www.ema.europa.eu/en/documents/scientific-guideline/questions-answers-allogeneic-stem-cell-based-products-veterinary-use-specific-questions-sterility_en.pdf (accessed February 15, 2020).
270. 270. FDA. *Veterinary Regenerative Medicine & Animal Cell-Based Products.* (2020). Available online at: https://www.fda.gov/animal-veterinary/development-approval-process/veterinary-regenerative-medicine-animal-cell-based-products~ (accessed February 15, 2020).
271. Caddeo S., Boffito M., Sartori S. Tissue Engineering Approaches in the Design of Healthy and Pathological In Vitro Tissue Models. *Front. Bioeng. Biotechnol.* 2017;5:40. doi: 10.3389/fbioe.2017.00040.
272. El-Husseiny H.M. *Master's Thesis.* Faculty of Veterinary Medicine, Benha University; Benha, Egypt: 2017. Evaluation of Some Prosthetic Implants for

Surgical Management of Different Varieties of Hernias in Domestic Animals; pp. 42–43.

273. El-Husseiny H.M., El-Maghraby H.M., Alakraa A.M., Kandiel M.M.M. Platelet Rich Fibrin Augmented Versus Non-Augmented Glycerolized Bovine Pericardium and Polypropylene Mesh for Repairing of Large Abdominal Wall Defects. *Eur. J. Med. Nat. Sci.* 2019;3:33–48. doi: 10.26417/767owa56e.

274. El-Husseiny H.M., Mady E.A., El-Dakroury W.A., Doghish A.S., Tanaka R. Stimuli-Responsive Hydrogels: Smart State of-the-Art Platforms for Cardiac Tissue Engineering. 2022. [(accessed on 10 September 2022)]. Available online: https://www.researchsquare.com/article/rs-2011475/v1

275. El-Husseiny H.M., Mady E.A., El-Dakroury W.A., Zewail M.B., Noshy M., Abdelfatah A.M., Doghish A.S. Smart/stimuli-responsive hydrogels: State-of-the-art platforms for bone tissue engineering. *Appl. Mater. Today.* 2022:101560. doi: 10.1016/j.apmt.2022.101560

276. El-Husseiny H.M., Mady E.A., Hamabe L., Abugomaa A., Shimada K., Yoshida T., Tanaka T., Yokoi A., Elbadawy M., Tanaka R. Smart/stimuli-responsive hydrogels: Cutting-edge platforms for tissue engineering and other biomedical applications. *Mater. Today Bio.* 2022;13:100186. doi: 10.1016/j.mtbio.2021.100186

277. Abd Elkodous M., El-Husseiny H.M., El-Sayyad G.S., Hashem A.H., Doghish A.S., Elfadil D., Radwan Y., El-Zeiny H.M., Bedair H., Ikhdair O.A., et al. Recent advances in waste-recycled nanomaterials for biomedical applications: Waste-to-wealth. *Nanotechnol. Rev.* 2021;10:1662–1739. doi: 10.1515/ntrev-2021-0099.

278. Dziubińska P., Jaskólska M., Przyborowska P., Adamiak Z. Stem cells in dentistry—Review of literature. *Pol. J. Vet. Sci.* 2013;16:135–140. doi: 10.2478/pjvs-2013-0021.

279. Hendawy H., Uemura A., Ma D., Namiki R., Samir H., Ahmed M.F., Elfadadny A., El-Husseiny H.M., Chieh-Jen C., Tanaka R. Tissue Harvesting Site Effect on the Canine Adipose Stromal Vascular Fraction Quantity and Quality. *Animals.* 2021;11:460. doi: 10.3390/ani11020460.

280. Ratajczak M., Zuba-Surma E., Ratajczak J. Stem Cell Therapeutics—Hope and Concerns. *Acta Haematol. Pol.* 2009;40:289–303. [Google Scholar]

281. Yamanaka S. Induced Pluripotent Stem Cells: Past, Present, and Future. *Cell Stem Cell.* 2012;10:678–684. doi: 10.1016/j.stem.2012.05.005.

282. Jayasuriya C.T., Hu N., Li J., Lemme N., Terek R., Ehrlich M.G., Chen Q. Molecular characterization of mesenchymal stem cells in human osteoarthritis cartilage reveals contribution to the OA phenotype. *Sci. Rep.* 2018;8:7044. doi: 10.1038/s41598-018-25395-8.

283. Frisbie D.D., Smith R.K.W. Clinical update on the use of mesenchymal stem cells in equine orthopaedics. *Equine Vet. J.* 2010;42:86–89. doi: 10.2746/042516409X477263.

284. Chopra H., Kumar Hans M., Shetty S. Stem cells-the hidden treasure: A strategic review. *Dent. Res. J.* 2013;10:421–427.

285. Krampera M., Franchini M., Pizzolo G., Aprili G. Mesenchymal stem cells: From biology to clinical use. *Blood Transfus.* 2007;5:120–129. doi: 10.2450/2007.0029-07.

286. Emura M. Stem cells of the respiratory epithelium and their in vitro cultivation. *Vitr. Cell. Dev. Biol.-Anim.* 1997;33:3–14. doi: 10.1007/s11626-997-0015-4.

287. Kolios G., Moodley Y. Introduction to Stem Cells and Regenerative Medicine. *Respiration.* 2013;85:3–10. doi: 10.1159/000345615.

288. Martin G.R. Isolation of a pluripotent cell line from early mouse embryos cultured in medium conditioned by teratocarcinoma stem cells. *Proc. Natl. Acad. Sci. USA.* 1981;78:7634–7638. doi: 10.1073/pnas.78.12.7634.

289. Evans M.J., Kaufman M.H. Establishment in culture of pluripotential cells from mouse embryos. *Nature.* 1981;292:154–156. doi: 10.1038/292154a0.

290. De Miguel M.P., Fuentes-Julián S., Alcaina Y. Pluripotent Stem Cells: Origin, Maintenance and Induction. *Stem Cell Rev. Rep.* 2010;6:633–649. doi: 10.1007/s12015-010-9170-1.

291. Guercio A., Di Marco P., Casella S., Cannella V., Russotto L., Purpari G., Di Bella S., Piccione G. Production of canine mesenchymal stem cells from adipose tissue and their application in dogs with chronic osteoarthritis of the humeroradial joints. *Cell Biol. Int.* 2012;36:189–194. doi: 10.1042/CBI20110304.

292. Nantavisai S., Egusa H., Osathanon T., Sawangmake C. Mesenchymal stem cell-based bone tissue engineering for veterinary practice. *Heliyon.* 2019;5:e02808. doi: 10.1016/j.heliyon.2019.e02808.

293. Augello A., Kurth T.B., De Bari C. Mesenchymal stem cells: A perspective from in vitro cultures to in vivo migration and niches. *Eur. Cells Mater.* 2010;20:e33. doi: 10.22203/eCM.v020a11.

294. Majo F., Rochat A., Nicolas M., Jaoudé G.A., Barrandon Y. Oligopotent stem cells are distributed throughout the mammalian ocular surface. *Nature.* 2008;456:250–254. doi: 10.1038/nature07406.

295. Burdzinska A., Idziak M. Stem Cells in Veterinary Medicine—Facts and Myths. *Mag. Weter.* 2013;7:695–704.

296. Voga M., Adamic N., Vengust M., Majdic G. Stem Cells in Veterinary Medicine—Current State and Treatment Options. *Front. Vet. Sci.* 2020;7:278. doi: 10.3389/fvets.2020.00278.
297. Takahashi K., Yamanaka S. Induction of Pluripotent Stem Cells from Mouse Embryonic and Adult Fibroblast Cultures by Defined Factors. *Cell.* 2006;126:663–676. doi: 10.1016/j.cell.2006.07.024.
298. Lin C.-S., Lin G., Lue T.F. Allogeneic and Xenogeneic Transplantation of Adipose-Derived Stem Cells in Immunocompetent Recipients Without Immunosuppressants. *Stem Cells Dev.* 2012;21:2770–2778. doi: 10.1089/scd.2012.0176.
299. Arzi B., Peralta S., Fiani N., Vapniarsky N., Taechangam N., Delatorre U., Clark K.C., Walker N.J., Loscar M.R., Lommer M.J., et al. A multicenter experience using adipose-derived mesenchymal stem cell therapy for cats with chronic, non-responsive gingivostomatitis. *Stem Cell Res. Ther.* 2020;11:115. doi: 10.1186/s13287-020-01623-9.
300. Kalisiak O., Cegielski M. Stem cells in treatment of tendon disorders in horses. *Życie Weter.* 2013;88:112–114.
301. Cegielski M., Kalisiak O. Stem Cells Therapy—A Hope For the Treatment of Tendons in Horses. *Życie Weter.* 2008;83:754–756. [Google Scholar]
302. Cegielski M., Izykowska I., Chmielewska M., Wojciech D., Bochnia M., Calkonski I., Dziegiel P. Characteristics of MIC-1 Antlerogenic Stem Cells and Their Effect on Hair Growth in Rabbits. *Vivo.* 2013;27:97–106.
303. Ding D.-C., Shyu W.-C., Lin S.-Z. Mesenchymal Stem Cells. *Cell Transplant.* 2011;20:5–14. doi: 10.3727/096368910X. [
304. Bearden R.N., Huggins S.S., Cummings K.J., Smith R., Gregory C.A., Saunders W.B. In-vitro characterization of canine multipotent stromal cells

isolated from synovium, bone marrow, and adipose tissue: A donor-matched comparative study. *Stem Cell Res. Ther.* 2017;8:218. doi: 10.1186/s13287-017-0639-6.

305. Godwin E.E., Young N.J., Dudhia J., Beamish I.C., Smith R.K.W. Implantation of bone marrow-derived mesenchymal stem cells demonstrates improved outcome in horses with overstrain injury of the superficial digital flexor tendon. *Equine Vet. J.* 2012;44:25–32. doi: 10.1111/j.2042-3306.2011.00363.x.
306. Peters A.E., Watts A.E. Biopsy Needle Advancement during Bone Marrow Aspiration Increases Mesenchymal Stem Cell Concentration. *Front. Vet. Sci.* 2016;3:23. doi: 10.3389/fvets.2016.00023.
307. Jacobs R.M., Kociba G.J., Ruoff W.W. Monoclonal Gammopathy in a Horse with Defective Hemostasis. *Vet. Pathol.* 1983;20:643–647. doi: 10.1177/030098588302000520.
308. Durando M.M., Zarucco L., Schaer T.P., Ross M., Reef V.B. Pneumopericardium in a horse secondary to sternal bone marrow aspiration. *Equine Vet. Educ.* 2006;18:75–79. doi: 10.1111/j.2042-3292.2006.tb00419.x.
309. Désévaux C., Laverty S., Doizé B. Sternal bone biopsy in standing horses. *Vet. Surg.* 2000;29:303–308.
310. Kasashima Y., Ueno T., Tomita A., Goodship A.E., Smith R.K.W. Optimisation of bone marrow aspiration from the equine sternum for the safe recovery of mesenchymal stem cells. *Equine Vet. J.* 2011;43:288–294. doi: 10.1111/j.2042-3306.2010.00215.x.
311. Rebelatto C.K., Aguiar A.M., Moretão M.P., Senegaglia A.C., Hansen P., Barchiki F., Oliveira J., Martins J., Kuligovski C., Mansur F., et al. Dissimilar

Differentiation of Mesenchymal Stem Cells from Bone Marrow, Umbilical Cord Blood, and Adipose Tissue. *Exp. Biol. Med.* 2008;233:901–913. doi: 10.3181/0712-RM-356.

312. Orbay H., Tobita M., Mizuno H. Mesenchymal Stem Cells Isolated from Adipose and Other Tissues: Basic Biological Properties and Clinical Applications. *Stem Cells Int.* 2012;2012:461718. doi: 10.1155/2012/461718.
313. Webb T.L., Quimby J.M., Dow S.W. In vitro comparison of feline bone marrow-derived and adipose tissue-derived mesenchymal stem cells. *J. Feline Med. Surg.* 2012;14:165–168. doi: 10.1177/1098612X11429224.
314. Cuervo B., Rubio M., Sopena J., Dominguez J.M., Vilar J., Morales M., Cugat R., Carrillo J.M. Hip Osteoarthritis in Dogs: A Randomized Study Using Mesenchymal Stem Cells from Adipose Tissue and Plasma Rich in Growth Factors. *Int. J. Mol. Sci.* 2014;15:13437–13460. doi: 10.3390/ijms150813437.
315. Vilar J.M., Morales M., Santana A., Spinella G., Rubio M., Cuervo B., Cugat R., Carrillo J.M. Controlled, blinded force platform analysis of the effect of intraarticular injection of autologous adipose-derived mesenchymal stem cells associated to PRGF-Endoret in osteoarthritic dogs. *BMC Vet. Res.* 2013;9:131. doi: 10.1186/1746-6148-9-131.
316. Koerner J., Nesic D., Romero J.D., Brehm W., Mainil-Varlet P., Grogan S.P. Equine Peripheral Blood-Derived Progenitors in Comparison to Bone Marrow-Derived Mesenchymal Stem Cells. *Stem Cells.* 2006;24:1613–1619. doi: 10.1634/stemcells.2005-0264.
317. Dhar M., Neilsen N., Beatty K., Eaker S., Adair H., Geiser D. Equine peripheral blood-derived mesenchymal stem cells: Isolation, identification,

trilineage differentiation and effect of hyperbaric oxygen treatment. *Equine Vet. J.* 2012;44:600–605. doi: 10.1111/j.2042-3306.2011.00536.x.

318. Spaas J.H., Schauwer C.D., Cornillie P., Meyer E., Soom A.V., Van de Walle G.R. Culture and characterisation of equine peripheral blood mesenchymal stromal cells. *Vet. J.* 2013;195:107–113. doi: 10.1016/j.tvjl.2012.05.006.
319. Chen M.Y., Lie P.C., Li Z.L., Wei X. Endothelial differentiation of Wharton's jelly-derived mesenchymal stem cells in comparison with bone marrow-derived mesenchymal stem cells. *Exp. Hematol.* 2009;37:629–640. doi: 10.1016/j.exphem.2009.02.003
320. In't Anker P.S., Scherjon S.A., Kleijburg-van der Keur C., de Groot-Swings G.M.J.S., Claas F.H.J., Fibbe W.E., Kanhai H.H.H. Isolation of Mesenchymal Stem Cells of Fetal or Maternal Origin from Human Placenta. *Stem Cells.* 2004;22:1338–1345. doi: 10.1634/stemcells.2004-0058.
321. Horse Embryonic Stem Cell Lines from the Proliferation of Inner Cell Mass Cells. *Stem Cells Dev.* 2006;15:523–531. doi: 10.1089/scd.2006.15.523.
322. Passeri S., Nocchi F., Lamanna R., Lapi S., Miragliotta V., Giannessi E., Abramo F., Stornelli M.R., Matarazzo M., Plenteda D., et al. Isolation and expansion of equine umbilical cord-derived matrix cells (EUCMCs) *Cell Biol. Int.* 2009;33:100–105. doi: 10.1016/j.cellbi.2008.10.012.
323. Prządka P., Kiełbowicz Z., Osiński B., Dzimira S., Madej J.A., Nowacki W., Kubiak K., Reichert P., Cegielski M. Reconstruction of cranial cruciate ligament in rabbits using polyester implants saturated with PRP, antlerogenic stem cells MIC-1 and their homogenate. *Connect. Tissue Res.* 2017;58:464–478. doi: 10.1080/03008207.2016.1251911.

324. Li C., Zhao H., Cheng L., Wang B. Allogeneic vs. autologous mesenchymal stem/stromal cells in their medication practice. *Cell Biosci.* 2021;11:187. doi: 10.1186/s13578-021-00698-y.
325. Penha E.M., Meira C.S., Guimarães E.T., Mendonça M.V.P., Gravely F.A., Pinheiro C.M.B., Pinheiro T.M.B., Barrouin-Melo S.M., Ribeiro-dos-Santos R., Soares M.B.P. Use of Autologous Mesenchymal Stem Cells Derived from Bone Marrow for the Treatment of Naturally Injured Spinal Cord in Dogs. *Stem Cells Int.* 2014;2014:437521. doi: 10.1155/2014/437521.
326. Feng M., Lu A., Gao H., Qian C., Zhang J., Lin T., Zhao Y. Safety of Allogeneic Umbilical Cord Blood Stem Cells Therapy in Patients with Severe Cerebral Palsy: A Retrospective Study. *Stem Cells Int.* 2015;2015:325652. doi: 10.1155/2015/325652.
327. Lee S.Y., Kim W., Lim C., Chung S.G. Treatment of Lateral Epicondylosis by Using Allogeneic Adipose-Derived Mesenchymal Stem Cells: A Pilot Study. *Stem Cells.* 2015;33:2995–3005. doi: 10.1002/stem.2110.
328. Sullivan M.J. Banking on cord blood stem cells. *Nat. Rev. Cancer.* 2008;8:555–563. doi: 10.1038/nrc2418.
329. Bertoni L., Branly T., Jacquet S., Desancé M., Desquilbet L., Rivory P., Hartmann D.-J., Denoix J.-M., Audigié F., Galéra P., et al. Intra-Articular Injection of 2 Different Dosages of Autologous and Allogeneic Bone Marrow- and Umbilical Cord-Derived Mesenchymal Stem Cells Triggers a Variable Inflammatory Response of the Fetlock Joint on 12 Sound Experimental Horses. *Stem Cells Int.* 2019;2019:9431894. doi: 10.1155/2019/9431894.
330. Prządka P., Buczak K., Frejlich E., Gąsior L., Suliga K., Kiełbowicz Z. The Role of Mesenchymal Stem Cells (MSCs) in Veterinary Medicine and Their

Use in Musculoskeletal Disorders. *Biomolecules.* 2021;11:1141. doi: 10.3390/biom11081141.

331. Devine S.M., Bartholomew A.M., Mahmud N., Nelson M., Patil S., Hardy W., Sturgeon C., Hewett T., Chung T., Stock W., et al. Mesenchymal stem cells are capable of homing to the bone marrow of non-human primates following systemic infusion. *Exp. Hematol.* 2001;29:244–255. doi: 10.1016/S0301-472X(00)00635-4.
332. Saito T., Kuang J.-Q., Bittira B., Al-Khaldi A., Chiu R.C.J. Xenotransplant cardiac chimera: Immune tolerance of adult stem cells. *Ann. Thorac. Surg.* 2002;74:19–24. doi: 10.1016/S0003-4975(02)03591-9.
333. Kim H.-J., Park J.-B., Lee J.K., Park E.-Y., Park E.-A., Riew K.D., Rhee S.-K. Transplanted xenogenic bone marrow stem cells survive and generate new bone formation in the posterolateral lumbar spine of non-immunosuppressed rabbits. *Eur. Spine J.* 2008;17:1515–1521. doi: 10.1007/s00586-008-0784-9.
334. Pal R., Gopinath C., Rao N.M., Banerjee P., Krishnamoorthy V., Venkataramana N.K., Totey S. Functional recovery after transplantation of bone marrow-derived human mesenchymal stromal cells in a rat model of spinal cord injury. *Cytotherapy.* 2010;12:792–806. doi: 10.3109/14653249.2010.487899.
335. Guan M., Yao W., Liu R., Lam K.S., Nolta J., Jia J., Panganiban B., Meng L., Zhou P., Shahnazari M., et al. Directing mesenchymal stem cells to bone to augment bone formation and increase bone mass. *Nat. Med.* 2012;18:456–462. doi: 10.1038/nm.2665.
336. Wieczorek M., Abualrous E.T., Sticht J., Álvaro-Benito M., Stolzenberg S., Noé F., Freund C. Major Histocompatibility Complex (MHC) Class I and

MHC Class II Proteins: Conformational Plasticity in Antigen Presentation. *Front. Immunol.* 2017;8:292. doi: 10.3389/fimmu.2017.00292.

337. Opiela J., Samiec M. Characterization of mesenchymal stem cells and their application in experimental embryology. *Pol. J. Vet. Sci.* 2013;16:593–599. doi: 10.2478/pjvs-2013-0084.

338. de Vasconcellos Machado C., da Silva Telles P.D., Nascimento I.L.O. Immunological characteristics of mesenchymal stem cells. *Rev. Bras. Hematol. E Hemoter.* 2013;35:62. doi: 10.5581/1516-8484.20130017.

339. Fortier L.A. Stem Cells: Classifications, Controversies, and Clinical Applications. *Vet. Surg.* 2005;34:415–423. doi: 10.1111/j.1532-950X.2005.00063.x.

340. Vizoso F.J., Eiro N., Cid S., Schneider J., Perez-Fernandez R. Mesenchymal Stem Cell Secretome: Toward Cell-Free Therapeutic Strategies in Regenerative Medicine. *Int. J. Mol. Sci.* 2017;18:1852. doi: 10.3390/ijms18091852.

341. Bari E., Ferrarotti I., Torre M.L., Corsico A.G., Perteghella S. Mesenchymal stem/stromal cell secretome for lung regeneration: The long way through “pharmaceuticalization” for the best formulation. *J. Control. Release.* 2019;309:11–24. doi: 10.1016/j.jconrel.2019.07.022.

342. El-Husseiny H., Mady E., Shimada K., Hamabe L., Yoshida T., Ma D., Mandour A., Hendawy H., Sasaki K., Fukuzumi S., et al. Intraventricular pressure gradient: A promising tool to predict the post-infarction chronic congestive heart failure in rats. *Eur. Heart J.-Cardiovasc. Imaging.* 2022;23:jeab289.390. doi: 10.1093/ehjci/jeab289.390.

343. El-Husseiny H.M., Mady E.A., Ma D., Hamabe L., Takahashi K., Tanaka R. Intraventricular pressure gradient: A novel tool to assess the post-infarction

chronic congestive heart failure. *Front. Cardiovasc. Med.* 2022;9:944717. doi: 10.3389/fcvm.2022.944171.

344. Ma D., Mandour A.S., Elfadadny A., Hendawy H., Yoshida T., El-Husseiny H.M., Nishifuji K., Takahashi K., Zhao Y., Zhou Z. Changes in cardiac function during the development of uremic cardiomyopathy and the effect of Salvianolic acid B administration in a rat model. *Front. Vet. Sci.* 2022;734:905759. doi: 10.3389/fvets.2022.905759.
345. Ma D., Mandour A.S., Hendawy H., Yoshida T., El-Husseiny H.M., Ozai Y., Takeuchi A., Takahashi K., Uemura A., Tanaka R. Renovascular Hypertension-Induced Cardiac Changes in a Rat Model: Feasibility Of Conventional And Recent Echocardiography. *J. Hypertens.* 2021;39:e403–e404. doi: 10.1097/01.hjh.0000749268.15046.a5.
346. Mandour A.S., Samir H., Yoshida T., Matsuura K., Abdelmageed H.A., Elbadawy M., Al-Rejaie S., El-Husseiny H.M., Elfadadny A., Ma D., et al. Assessment of the Cardiac Functions Using Full Conventional Echocardiography with Tissue Doppler Imaging before and after Xylazine Sedation in Male Shiba Goats. *Animals.* 2020;10:2320. doi: 10.3390/ani10122320.
347. Sasaki K., Ma D., Mandour A.S., Ozai Y., Yoshida T., Matsuura K., Takeuchi A., Cheng C.-J., El-Husseiny H.M., Hendawy H., et al. Evaluation of Changes in the Cardiac Function before and after Transcatheter Edge-to-Edge Mitral Valve Repair in Healthy Dogs: Conventional and Novel Echocardiography. *Animals.* 2022;12:56. doi: 10.3390/ani12010056.
348. Yairo A., Mandour A.S., Matsuura K., Yoshida T., Ma D., Kitpipatkun P., Kato K., Cheng C.-J., El-Husseiny H.M., Tanaka T., et al. Effect of Loading Changes on the Intraventricular Pressure Measured by Color M-Mode

Echocardiography in Rats. *Diagnostics.* 2021;11:1403. doi: 10.3390/diagnostics11081403.

349. Yoshida T., Mandour A.S., Matsuura K., Shimada K., El-Husseiny H.M., Hamabe L., Yilmaz Z., Uemura A., Tanaka R. Changes in the Pulmonary Artery Wave Reflection in Dogs with Experimentally-Induced Acute Pulmonary Embolism and the Effect of Vasodilator. *Animals.* 2021;11:1977. doi: 10.3390/ani11071977.
350. Yoshida T., Matsuura K., Chieh-Jen C., Aboshi Y., Yamada S., Yotsuida H., Hasegawa M., Hendawy H.A., El-Husseiny H.M., Takahashi Y., et al. Surgical treatment for left atrial rupture due to myxomatous mitral valve disease in three dogs: A case report. *Vet. Med. Sci.* 2022:1–7. doi: 10.1002/vms3.915.
351. Hamabe L., Shimada K., Mandour A.S., Yoshida T., Hirose M., Hendawy H., El-Husseiny H.M., Tanaka R. Evaluation of Left Ventricular Function in Healthy Retrievers Using Standard and 2D Speckle-Tracking Echocardiography. *Vet. Sci.* 2022;9:529. doi: 10.3390/vetsci9100529.
352. Pogue B., Estrada A.H., Sosa-Samper I., Maisenbacher H.W., Lamb K.E., Mincey B.D., Erger K.E., Conlon T.J. Stem-cell therapy for dilated cardiomyopathy: A pilot study evaluating retrograde coronary venous delivery. *J. Small Anim. Pract.* 2013;54:361–366. doi: 10.1111/jsap.12098.
353. Hensley M.T., Tang J., Woodruff K., Defrancesco T., Tou S., Williams C.M., Breen M., Meurs K., Keene B., Cheng K. Intracoronary allogeneic cardiosphere-derived stem cells are safe for use in dogs with dilated cardiomyopathy. *J. Cell. Mol. Med.* 2017;21:1503–1512. doi: 10.1111/jcmm.13077.

354. Petchdee S., Sompeewong S. Intravenous administration of puppy deciduous teeth stem cells in degenerative valve disease. *Vet. World.* 2016;9:1429. doi: 10.14202/vetworld.2016.1429-1434.

355. Pratheesh M.D., Dubey P.K., Gade N.E., Nath A., Sivanarayanan T.B., Madhu D.N., Somal A., Baiju I., Sreekumar T.R., Gleeja V.L., et al. Comparative study on characterization and wound healing potential of goat (*Capra hircus*) mesenchymal stem cells derived from fetal origin amniotic fluid and adult bone marrow. *Res. Vet. Sci.* 2017;112:81–88. doi: 10.1016/j.rvsc.2016.12.009.

356. Martinello T., Gomiero C., Perazzi A., Iacopetti I., Gemignani F., DeBenedictis G.M., Ferro S., Zuin M., Martines E., Brun P., et al. Allogeneic mesenchymal stem cells improve the wound healing process of sheep skin. *BMC Vet. Res.* 2018;14:202. doi: 10.1186/s12917-018-1527-8.

357. Textor J.A., Clark K.C., Walker N.J., Aristizobal F.A., Kol A., LeJeune S.S., Bledsoe A., Davidyan A., Gray S.N., Bohannon-Worsley L.K., et al. Allogeneic Stem Cells Alter Gene Expression and Improve Healing of Distal Limb Wounds in Horses. *Stem Cells Transl. Med.* 2017;7:98–108. doi: 10.1002/sctm.17-0071

358. Venkataiah V.S., Handa K., Njuguna M.M., Hasegawa T., Maruyama K., Nemoto E., Yamada S., Sugawara S., Lu L., Takedachi M., et al. Periodontal Regeneration by Allogeneic Transplantation of Adipose Tissue Derived Multi-Lineage Progenitor Stem Cells in vivo. *Sci. Rep.* 2019;9:921. doi: 10.1038/s41598-018-37528-0.

359. Abdelaz P., ElZoghbi A., Shokry M., Ahmed A.-Z., Rasha H. Reparative dentin formation using stem cell therapy versus calcium hydroxide in direct

pulp capping: An animal study. *Braz. Dent. J.* 2019;30:542–549. doi: 10.1590/0103-6440201902711.

360. Iohara K., Utsunomiya S., Kohara S., Nakashima M. Allogeneic transplantation of mobilized dental pulp stem cells with the mismatched dog leukocyte antigen type is safe and efficacious for total pulp regeneration. *Stem Cell Res. Ther.* 2018;9:116. doi: 10.1186/s13287-018-0855-8.]

361. Pérez-Merino E.M., Usón-Casaús J.M., Duque-Carrasco J., Zaragoza-Bayle C., Mariñas-Pardo L., Hermida-Prieto M., Vilafranca-Compte M., Barrera-Chacón R., Gualtieri M. Safety and efficacy of allogeneic adipose tissue-derived mesenchymal stem cells for treatment of dogs with inflammatory bowel disease: Endoscopic and histological outcomes. *Vet. J.* 2015;206:391–397. doi: 10.1016/j.tvjl.2015.07.023.

362. Webb T.L., Webb C.B. Stem cell therapy in cats with chronic enteropathy: A proof-of-concept study. *J. Feline Med. Surg.* 2015;17:901–908. doi: 10.1177/1098612X14561105.

363. Yan Y., Fang J., Wen X., Teng X., Li B., Zhou Z., Peng S., Arisha A.H., Liu W., Hua J. Therapeutic applications of adipose-derived mesenchymal stem cells on acute liver injury in canines. *Res. Vet. Sci.* 2019;126:233–239. doi: 10.1016/j.rvsc.2019.09.004.

364. Matsuda T., Takami T., Sasaki R., Nishimura T., Aibe Y., Paredes B.D., Quintanilha L.F., Matsumoto T., Ishikawa T., Yamamoto N., et al. A canine liver fibrosis model to develop a therapy for liver cirrhosis using cultured bone marrow–derived cells. *Hepatol. Commun.* 2017;1:691–703. doi: 10.1002/hep4.1071.

365. Renzi S., Riccò S., Dotti S., Sesso L., Grolli S., Cornali M., Carlin S., Patruno M., Cinotti S., Ferrari M. Autologous bone marrow mesenchymal stromal

cells for regeneration of injured equine ligaments and tendons: A clinical report. *Res. Vet. Sci.* 2013;95:272–277. doi: 10.1016/j.rvsc.2013.01.017.

366. Smith R.K.W., Korda M., Blunn G.W., Goodship A.E. Isolation and implantation of autologous equine mesenchymal stem cells from bone marrow into the superficial digital flexor tendon as a potential novel treatment. *Equine Vet. J.* 2003;35:99–102. doi: 10.2746/042516403775467388.
367. Ferris D.J., Frisbie D.D., Kisiday J.D., McIlwraith C.W., Hague B.A., Major M.D., Schneider R.K., Zubrod C.J., Kawcak C.E., Goodrich L.R. Clinical Outcome After Intra-Articular Administration of Bone Marrow Derived Mesenchymal Stem Cells in 33 Horses With Stifle Injury. *Vet. Surg.* 2014;43:255–265. doi: 10.1111/j.1532-950X.2014.12100.x.
368. Mariñas-Pardo L., Rodríguez-Hurtado I., Rodríguez-García M.I., Núñez-Naveira L., Hermida-Prieto M. Allogeneic Adipose-Derived Mesenchymal Stem Cells (Horse Allo 20) for the Treatment of Osteoarthritis-Associated Lameness in Horses: Characterization, Safety, and Efficacy of Intra-Articular Treatment. *Stem Cells Dev.* 2018;27:1147–1160. doi: 10.1089/scd.2018.0074.
369. Besalti O., Aktas Z., Can P., Akpinar E., Elcin A.E., Elcin Y.M. The use of autologous neurogenically-induced bone marrow-derived mesenchymal stem cells for the treatment of paraplegic dogs without nociception due to spinal trauma. *J. Vet. Med. Sci.* 2016;78:1465–1473. doi: 10.1292/jvms.15-0571.
370. Bhat I.A., Sivanarayanan T.B., Somal A., Pandey S., Bharti M.K., Panda B.S., Verma M., Sonwane A., Kumar G.S., Chandra V., et al. An allogenic therapeutic strategy for canine spinal cord injury using mesenchymal stem cells. *J. Cell. Physiol.* 2019;234:2705–2718. doi: 10.1002/jcp.27086.

371. Quimby J.M., Webb T.L., Gibbons D.S., Dow S.W. Evaluation of intrarenal mesenchymal stem cell injection for treatment of chronic kidney disease in cats: A pilot study. *J. Feline Med. Surg.* 2011;13:418–426. doi: 10.1016/j.jfms.2011.01.005.
372. Vidane A.S., Pinheiro A.O., Casals J.B., Passarelli D., Hage M., Bueno R.S., Martins D.S., Ambrósio C.E. Transplantation of amniotic membrane-derived multipotent cells ameliorates and delays the progression of chronic kidney disease in cats. *Reprod. Domest. Anim.* 2017;52:316–326. doi: 10.1111/rda.12846.
373. Barussi F.C.M., Bastos F.Z., Leite L.M.B., Fragoso F.Y.I., Senegaglia A.C., Brofman P.R.S., Nishiyama A., Pimpão C.T., Michelotto P.V. Intratracheal therapy with autologous bone marrow-derived mononuclear cells reduces airway inflammation in horses with recurrent airway obstruction. *Respir. Physiol. Neurobiol.* 2016;232:35–42. doi: 10.1016/j.resp.2016.07.002.
374. Hao Y., Ran Y., Lu B., Li J., Zhang J., Feng C., Fang J., Ma R., Qiao Z., Dai X., et al. Therapeutic Effects of Human Umbilical Cord–Derived Mesenchymal Stem Cells on Canine Radiation-Induced Lung Injury. *Int. J. Radiat. Oncol. Biol. Phys.* 2018;102:407–416. doi: 10.1016/j.ijrobp.2018.05.068.
375. Davis A.B., Schnabel L.V., Gilger B.C. Subconjunctival bone marrow-derived mesenchymal stem cell therapy as a novel treatment alternative for equine immune-mediated keratitis: A case series. *Vet. Ophthalmol.* 2019;22:674–682. doi: 10.1111/vop.12641.
376. Villatoro A.J., Claros S., Fernández V., Alcoholado C., Fariñas F., Moreno A., Becerra J., Andrades J.A. Safety and efficacy of the mesenchymal stem

cell in feline eosinophilic keratitis treatment. *BMC Vet. Res.* 2018;14:116. doi: 10.1186/s12917-018-1413-4.

377. Wernly B., Mirna M., Rezar R., Prodinger C., Jung C., Podesser B.K., Kiss A., Hoppe U.C., Lichtenauer M. Regenerative Cardiovascular Therapies: Stem Cells and Beyond. *Int. J. Mol. Sci.* 2019;20:1420. doi: 10.3390/ijms20061420

378. Hoffman A.M., Dow S.W. Concise Review: Stem Cell Trials Using Companion Animal Disease Models. *Stem Cells.* 2016;34:1709–1729. doi: 10.1002/stem.2377.

379. Fox P.R. Pathology of myxomatous mitral valve disease in the dog. *J. Vet. Cardiol.* 2012;14:103–126. doi: 10.1016/j.jvc.2012.02.001.

380. Ojeh N., Pastar I., Tomic-Canic M., Stojadinovic O. Stem Cells in Skin Regeneration, Wound Healing, and Their Clinical Applications. *Int. J. Mol. Sci.* 2015;16:25476–25501. doi: 10.3390/ijms161025476.

381. Johnson V., Webb T., Norman A., Coy J., Kurihara J., Regan D., Dow S. Activated Mesenchymal Stem Cells Interact with Antibiotics and Host Innate Immune Responses to Control Chronic Bacterial Infections. *Sci. Rep.* 2017;7:9575. doi: 10.1038/s41598-017-08311-4.]

382. El-Tookhy O.S., Shamaa A.A., Shehab G.G., Abdallah A.N., Azzam O.M. Histological Evaluation of Experimentally Induced Critical Size Defect Skin Wounds Using Exosomal Solution of Mesenchymal Stem Cells Derived Microvesicles. *Int. J. Stem Cells.* 2017;10:144–153. doi: 10.15283/ijsc17043.

383. Spaas J.H., Broeckx S., Van de Walle G.R., Polettini M. The effects of equine peripheral blood stem cells on cutaneous wound healing: A clinical evaluation in four horses. *Clin. Exp. Dermatol.* 2013;38:280–284. doi: 10.1111/ced.12068.

384. Lanci A., Merlo B., Mariella J., Castagnetti C., Iacono E. Heterologous Wharton's Jelly Derived Mesenchymal Stem Cells Application on a Large Chronic Skin Wound in a 6-Month-Old Filly. *Front. Vet. Sci.* 2019;6:9. doi: 10.3389/fvets.2019.00009.
385. Hall M., Rosenkrantz W.S., Hong J., Griffin C.E., Mendelsohn C. Evaluation of the potential use of adipose-derived mesenchymal stromal cells in the treatment of canine atopic dermatitis: A pilot study. *Vet. Ther.* 2010;11:E1–E14.
386. Villatoro A.J., Hermida-Prieto M., Fernández V., Fariñas F., Alcoholado C., Rodríguez-García M.I., Mariñas-Pardo L., Becerra J. Allogeneic adipose-derived mesenchymal stem cell therapy in dogs with refractory atopic dermatitis: Clinical efficacy and safety. *Vet. Rec.* 2018;183:654. doi: 10.1136/vr.104867.
387. Babu N.C., Gomes A.J. Systemic manifestations of oral diseases. *J. Oral Maxillofac. Pathol.* 2011;15:144. doi: 10.4103/0973-029X.84477.
388. Javdani M., Nikousefat Z. Prevalence of dental problems in pet dogs in Shiraz, Iran Res. *Opin. Anim. Vet. Sci.* 2011;1:666–668.
389. Niemiec B., Gawor J., Nemec A., Clarke D., McLeod K., Tutt C., Gioso M., Steagall P.V., Chandler M., Morgenegg G., et al. World Small Animal Veterinary Association Global Dental Guidelines. *J. Small Anim. Pract.* 2020;61:E36–E161. doi: 10.1111/jsap.13132.
390. El-Zekrid M.H., Mahmoud S.H., Ali F.A., Helal M.E., Grawish M.E. Healing Capacity of Autologous Bone Marrow–derived Mesenchymal Stem Cells on Partially Pulpotomized Dogs' Teeth. *J. Endod.* 2019;45:287–294. doi: 10.1016/j.joen.2018.11.013.

391. Sánchez-Garcés M.À., Alvira-González J., Sánchez C.M., Cairó J.R.B., Del Pozo M.R., Gay-Escoda C. Bone Regeneration Using Adipose-Derived Stem Cells with Fibronectin in Dehiscence-Type Defects Associated with Dental Implants: An Experimental Study in a Dog Model. *Int. J. Oral Maxillofac. Implant.* 2017;32:e97–e106. doi: 10.11607/jomi.5169.
392. Bellei E., Dalla F., Masetti L., Pisoni L., Joechler M. Surgical therapy in chronic feline gingivostomatitis (FCGS) *Vet. Res. Commun.* 2008;32:231–234. doi: 10.1007/s11259-008-9153-8.
393. Hennet P.R., Camy G.A.L., McGahie D.M., Albouy M.V. Comparative efficacy of a recombinant feline interferon omega in refractory cases of calicivirus-positive cats with caudal stomatitis: A randomised, multi-centre, controlled, double-blind study in 39 cats. *J. Feline Med. Surg.* 2011;13:577–587. doi: 10.1016/j.jfms.2011.05.012
394. Lommer M.J. Efficacy of Cyclosporine for Chronic, Refractory Stomatitis in Cats: A Randomized, Placebo-Controlled, Double-Blinded Clinical Study. *J. Vet. Dent.* 2013;30:8–17. doi: 10.1177/089875641303000101.
395. Druet I., Hennet P. Relationship between Feline calicivirus Load, Oral Lesions, and Outcome in Feline Chronic Gingivostomatitis (Caudal Stomatitis): Retrospective Study in 104 Cats. *Front. Vet. Sci.* 2017;4:209. doi: 10.3389/fvets.2017.00209.
396. Winer J.N., Arzi B., Verstraete F.J.M. Therapeutic Management of Feline Chronic Gingivostomatitis: A Systematic Review of the Literature. *Front. Vet. Sci.* 2016;3:54. doi: 10.3389/fvets.2016.00054.
397. Arzi B., Mills-Ko E., Verstraete F.J.M., Kol A., Walker N.J., Badgley M.R., Fazel N., Murphy W.J., Vapniarsky N., Borjesson D.L. Therapeutic Efficacy of Fresh, Autologous Mesenchymal Stem Cells for Severe Refractory

Gingivostomatitis in Cats. *Stem Cells Transl. Med.* 2015;5:75–86. doi: 10.5966/sctm.2015-0127.

398. Arzi B., Clark K.C., Sundaram A., Spriet M., Verstraete F.J.M., Walker N.J., Loscar M.R., Fazel N., Murphy W.J., Vapniarsky N., et al. Therapeutic Efficacy of Fresh, Allogeneic Mesenchymal Stem Cells for Severe Refractory Feline Chronic Gingivostomatitis. *Stem Cells Transl. Med.* 2017;6:1710–1722. doi: 10.1002/sctm.17-0035.
399. Craven M., Simpson J.W., Ridyard A.E., Chandler M.L. Canine inflammatory bowel disease: Retrospective analysis of diagnosis and outcome in 80 cases (1995–2002) *J. Small Anim. Pract.* 2004;45:336–342. doi: 10.1111/j.1748-5827.2004.tb00245.x
400. Hall E.J. *Inflammatory Bowel Disease in Dogs and Cats.* Hill's Pet Nutrition, Inc.; Topeka, KS, USA: 2009. [(accessed on 10 September 2022)]. Available online: https://protrain.hs.llnwd.net/e1/sitefiles/642/Documents/GI%20technical%20booklet.pdf]
401. Nishimura T., Takami T., Sasaki R., Aibe Y., Matsuda T., Fujisawa K., Matsumoto T., Yamamoto N., Tani K., Taura Y., et al. Liver regeneration therapy through the hepatic artery-infusion of cultured bone marrow cells in a canine liver fibrosis model. *PLoS ONE.* 2019;14:e0210588. doi: 10.1371/journal.pone.0210588
402. Gardin C., Ferroni L., Bellin G., Rubini G., Barosio S., Zavan B. Therapeutic Potential of Autologous Adipose-Derived Stem Cells for the Treatment of Liver Disease. *Int. J. Mol. Sci.* 2018;19:4064. doi: 10.3390/ijms19124064.
403. Nam A., Han S.M., Go D.M., Kim D.Y., Seo K.W., Youn H.Y. Long-Term Management with Adipose Tissue-Derived Mesenchymal Stem Cells and

Conventional Treatment in a Dog with Hepatocutaneous Syndrome. *J. Vet. Intern. Med.* 2017;31:1514–1519. doi: 10.1111/jvim.14798.

404. de Witte S.F.H., Luk F., Sierra Parraga J.M., Gargesha M., Merino A., Korevaar S.S., Shankar A.S., O'Flynn L., Elliman S.J., Roy D., et al. Immunomodulation By Therapeutic Mesenchymal Stromal Cells (MSC) Is Triggered Through Phagocytosis of MSC By Monocytic Cells. *Stem Cells.* 2018;36:602–615. doi: 10.1002/stem.2779.
405. Dakin S.G., Jespers K., Warner S., O'hara L.K., Dudhia J., Goodship A.E., Wilson A.M., Smith R.K.W. The relationship between in vivo limb and in vitro tendon mechanics after injury: A potential novel clinical tool for monitoring tendon repair. *Equine Vet. J.* 2011;43:418–423. doi: 10.1111/j.2042-3306.2010.00303.x.
406. Petrov R., MacDonald M.H., Tesch A.M., Hoogmoed L.M.V. Influence of topically applied cold treatment on core temperature and cell viability in equine superficial digital flexor tendons. *Am. J. Vet. Res.* 2003;64:835–844. doi: 10.2460/ajvr.2003.64.835.
407. Chan K.-M., Fu S.-C. Anti-inflammatory management for tendon injuries-friends or foes? *BMC Sport. Sci. Med. Rehabil.* 2009;1:23. doi: 10.1186/1758-2555-1-23.
408. Eliashar E., Schramme M.C., Schumacher J., Smith R.K.W., Ikada Y. Use of a bioabsorbable implant for the repair of severed digital flexor tendons in four horses. *Vet. Rec.* 2001;148:506–509. doi: 10.1136/vr.148.16.506.
409. Filomeno P., Dayan V., Touriño C. Stem cell research and clinical development in tendon repair. *Muscles Ligaments Tendons J.* 2012;2:204.

410. Costa-Almeida R., Calejo I., Gomes M.E. Mesenchymal Stem Cells Empowering Tendon Regenerative Therapies. *Int. J. Mol. Sci.* 2019;20:3002. doi: 10.3390/ijms20123002.
411. Pacini S., Spinabella S., Trombi L., Fazzi R., Galimberti S., Dini F., Carlucci F., Petrini M. Suspension of Bone Marrow–Derived Undifferentiated Mesenchymal Stromal Cells for Repair of Superficial Digital Flexor Tendon in Race Horses. *Tissue Eng.* 2007;13:2949–2955. doi: 10.1089/ten.2007.0108.
412. Dyson S.J. Medical management of superficial digital flexor tendonitis: A comparative study in 219 horses (1992–2000) *Equine Vet. J.* 2004;36:415–419. doi: 10.2746/0425164044868422.
413. Smith R.K.W., Werling N.J., Dakin S.G., Alam R., Goodship A.E., Dudhia J. Beneficial Effects of Autologous Bone Marrow-Derived Mesenchymal Stem Cells in Naturally Occurring Tendinopathy. *PLoS ONE.* 2013;8:e75697. doi: 10.1371/annotation/a30a4b87-8904-4510-b0a8-5b6ca6097f9a.
414. Van Loon V.J.F., Scheffer C.J.W., Genn H.J., Hoogendoorn A.C., Greve J.W. Clinical follow-up of horses treated with allogeneic equine mesenchymal stem cells derived from umbilical cord blood for different tendon and ligament disorders. *Vet. Q.* 2014;34:92–97. doi: 10.1080/01652176.2014.949390.
415. Romero A., Barrachina L., Ranera B., Remacha A.R., Moreno B., de Blas I., Sanz A., Vázquez F.J., Vitoria A., Junquera C., et al. Comparison of autologous bone marrow and adipose tissue derived mesenchymal stem cells, and platelet rich plasma, for treating surgically induced lesions of the equine superficial digital flexor tendon. *Vet. J.* 2017;224:76–84. doi: 10.1016/j.tvjl.2017.04.005.

416. Geburek F., Roggel F., van Schie H.T.M., Beineke A., Estrada R., Weber K., Hellige M., Rohn K., Jagodzinski M., Welke B., et al. Effect of single intralesional treatment of surgically induced equine superficial digital flexor tendon core lesions with adipose-derived mesenchymal stromal cells: A controlled experimental trial. *Stem Cell Res. Ther.* 2017;8:129. doi: 10.1186/s13287-017-0564-8

417. Harasen G. Diagnosing rupture of the cranial cruciate ligament. *Can. Vet. J.* 2002;43:475.

418. Chuang C., Ramaker M.A., Kaur S., Csomos R.A., Kroner K.T., Bleedorn J.A., Schaefer S.L., Muir P. Radiographic Risk Factors for Contralateral Rupture in Dogs with Unilateral Cranial Cruciate Ligament Rupture. *PLoS ONE.* 2014;9:e106389. doi: 10.1371/journal.pone.0106389.

419. Mölsä S.H., Hyytiäinen H.K., Hielm-Björkman A.K., Laitinen-Vapaavuori O.M. Long-term functional outcome after surgical repair of cranial cruciate ligament disease in dogs. *BMC Vet. Res.* 2014;10:266. doi: 10.1186/s12917-014-0266-8.

420. Taroni M., Cabon Q., Fèbre M., Cachon T., Saulnier N., Carozzo C., Maddens S., Labadie F., Robert C., Viguier E. Evaluation of the Effect of a Single Intra-articular Injection of Allogeneic Neonatal Mesenchymal Stromal Cells Compared to Oral Non-Steroidal Anti-inflammatory Treatment on the Postoperative Musculoskeletal Status and Gait of Dogs over a 6-Month Period after Tibial Plateau Leveling Osteotomy: A Pilot Study. *Front. Vet. Sci.* 2017;4:83. doi: 10.3389/fvets.2017.00083.

421. Linon E., Spreng D., Rytz U., Forterre S. Engraftment of autologous bone marrow cells into the injured cranial cruciate ligament in dogs. *Vet. J.* 2014;202:448–454. doi: 10.1016/j.tvjl.2014.08.031.

422. Muir P., Hans E.C., Racette M., Volstad N., Sample S.J., Heaton C., Holzman G., Schaefer S.L., Bloom D.D., Bleedorn J.A., et al. Autologous Bone Marrow-Derived Mesenchymal Stem Cells Modulate Molecular Markers of Inflammation in Dogs with Cruciate Ligament Rupture. *PLoS ONE.* 2016;11:e0159095. doi: 10.1371/journal.pone.0159095.
423. Canapp S.O., Leasure C.S., Cox C., Ibrahim V., Carr B.J. Partial Cranial Cruciate Ligament Tears Treated with Stem Cell and Platelet-Rich Plasma Combination Therapy in 36 Dogs: A Retrospective Study. *Front. Vet. Sci.* 2016;3:112. doi: 10.3389/fvets.2016.00112.
424. Frisbie D.D., Stewart M.C. Cell-based Therapies for Equine Joint Disease. *Vet. Clin. N. Am. Equine Pract.* 2011;27:335–349. doi: 10.1016/j.cveq.2011.06.005.
425. Rossdale P., Hopes R., Digby N. Epidemiological study of wastage among racehorses 1982 and 1983. *Vet. Rec.* 1985;116:66–69. doi: 10.1136/vr.116.3.66.
426. Walmsley J.P., Phillips T.J., Townsend H.G.G. Meniscal tears in horses: An evaluation of clinical signs and arthroscopic treatment of 80 cases. *Equine Vet. J.* 2003;35:402–406. doi: 10.2746/042516403776014163.
427. Nicpoń J., Marycz K., Grzesiak J. Therapeutic effect of adipose-derived mesenchymal stem cell injection in horses suffering from bone spavin. *Pol. J. Vet. Sci.* 2013;16:753–754. doi: 10.2478/pjvs-2013-0107.]
428. Joswig A.-J., Mitchell A., Cummings K.J., Levine G.J., Gregory C.A., Smith R., Watts A.E. Repeated intra-articular injection of allogeneic mesenchymal stem cells causes an adverse response compared to autologous cells in the equine model. *Stem Cell Res. Ther.* 2017;8:42. doi: 10.1186/s13287-017-0503-8.

429. Mohoric L., Zorko B., Ceh K., Majdic G. Blinded placebo study of bilateral osteoarthritis treatment using adipose derived mesenchymal stem cells. *Slov. Vet. Res.* 2016;53:167–174.

430. Black L.L., Gaynor J., Gahring D., Adams C., Aron D., Harman S., Gingerich D.A., Harman R. Effect of adipose-derived mesenchymal stem and regenerative cells on lameness in dogs with chronic osteoarthritis of the coxofemoral joints: A randomized, double-blinded, multicenter controlled trial. *Vet. Ther.* 2007;8:272

431. Srzentić Dražilov S., Mrkovački J., Spasovski V., Fazlagić A., Pavlović S., Nikčević G. The use of canine mesenchymal stem cells for the autologous treatment of osteoarthritis. *Acta Vet. Hung.* 2018;66:376–389. doi: 10.1556/004.2018.034.

432. Harman R., Carlson K., Gaynor J., Gustafson S., Dhupa S., Clement K., Hoelzler M., McCarthy T., Schwartz P., Adams C. A Prospective, Randomized, Masked, and Placebo-Controlled Efficacy Study of Intraarticular Allogeneic Adipose Stem Cells for the Treatment of Osteoarthritis in Dogs. *Front. Vet. Sci.* 2016;3:81. doi: 10.3389/fvets.2016.00081.

433. Shah K., Drury T., Roic I., Hansen P., Malin M., Boyd R., Sumer H., Ferguson R. Outcome of Allogeneic Adult Stem Cell Therapy in Dogs Suffering from Osteoarthritis and Other Joint Defects. *Stem Cells Int.* 2018;2018:7309201. doi: 10.1155/2018/7309201.

434. Zhang B.-y., Wang B.-y., Li S.-c., Luo D.-z., Zhan X., Chen S.-f., Chen Z.-s., Liu C.-y., Ji H.-q., Bai Y.-s., et al. Evaluation of the Curative Effect of Umbilical Cord Mesenchymal Stem Cell Therapy for Knee Arthritis in Dogs

Using Imaging Technology. *Stem Cells Int.* 2018;2018:1983025. doi: 10.1155/2018/1983025.

435. Cabon Q., Febre M., Gomez N., Cachon T., Pillard P., Carozzo C., Saulnier N., Robert C., Livet V., Rakic R., et al. Long-Term Safety and Efficacy of Single or Repeated Intra-Articular Injection of Allogeneic Neonatal Mesenchymal Stromal Cells for Managing Pain and Lameness in Moderate to Severe Canine Osteoarthritis Without Anti-inflammatory Pharmacological Support: Pilot Clinical Study. *Front. Vet. Sci.* 2019;6:10. doi: 10.3389/fvets.2019.00010.

436. Li L., Duan X., Fan Z., Chen L., Xing F., Xu Z., Chen Q., Xiang Z. Mesenchymal Stem Cells in Combination with Hyaluronic Acid for Articular Cartilage Defects. *Sci. Rep.* 2018;8:9900. doi: 10.1038/s41598-018-27737-y.

437. Kornicka-Garbowska K., Pędziwiatr R., Woźniak P., Kucharczyk K., Marycz K. Microvesicles isolated from 5-azacytidine-and-resveratrol-treated mesenchymal stem cells for the treatment of suspensory ligament injury in horse—A case report. *Stem Cell Res. Ther.* 2019;10:394. doi: 10.1186/s13287-019-1469-5

438. Bach F.S., Rebelatto C.L.K., Fracaro L., Senegaglia A.C., Fragoso F.Y.I., Daga D.R., Brofman P.R.S., Pimpão C.T., Engracia Filho J.R., Montiani-Ferreira F., et al. Comparison of the Efficacy of Surgical Decompression Alone and Combined With Canine Adipose Tissue-Derived Stem Cell Transplantation in Dogs With Acute Thoracolumbar Disk Disease and Spinal Cord Injury. *Front. Vet. Sci.* 2019;6:383. doi: 10.3389/fvets.2019.00383.

439. Bone Marrow-Derived Mesenchymal Stem Cells as Autologous Therapy in Dogs with Naturally Occurring Intervertebral Disc Disease: Feasibility,

Safety, and Preliminary Results. *Tissue Eng. Part C Methods.* 2017;23:643–651. doi: 10.1089/ten.tec.2017.0033.

440. Wu G.-H., Shi H.-J., Che M.-T., Huang M.-Y., Wei Q.-S., Feng B., Ma Y.-H., Wang L.-J., Jiang B., Wang Y.-Q., et al. Recovery of paralyzed limb motor function in canine with complete spinal cord injury following implantation of MSC-derived neural network tissue. *Biomaterials.* 2018;181:15–34. doi: 10.1016/j.biomaterials.2018.07.010.
441. Adin C.A., Gregory C.R., Kyles A.E., Cowgill L. Diagnostic Predictors of Complications and Survival after Renal Transplantation in Cats. *Vet. Surg.* 2001;30:515–521. doi: 10.1053/jvet.2001.28418.
442. Quimby J.M., Webb T.L., Habenicht L.M., Dow S.W. Safety and efficacy of intravenous infusion of allogeneic cryopreserved mesenchymal stem cells for treatment of chronic kidney disease in cats: Results of three sequential pilot studies. *Stem Cell Res. Ther.* 2013;4:48. doi: 10.1186/scrt198.
443. Quimby J.M., Webb T.L., Randall E., Marolf A., Valdes-Martinez A., Dow S.W. Assessment of intravenous adipose-derived allogeneic mesenchymal stem cells for the treatment of feline chronic kidney disease: A randomized, placebo-controlled clinical trial in eight cats. *J. Feline Med. Surg.* 2016;18:165–171. doi: 10.1177/1098612X15576980.
444. Trzil J.E., Masseau I., Webb T.L., Chang C.-H., Dodam J.R., Liu H., Quimby J.M., Dow S.W., Reinero C.R. Intravenous adipose-derived mesenchymal stem cell therapy for the treatment of feline asthma: A pilot study. *J. Feline Med. Surg.* 2016;18:981–990. doi: 10.1177/1098612X15604351.]
445. Marfe G., Massaro-Giordano M., Ranalli M., Cozzoli E., Di Stefano C., Malafoglia V., Polettini M., Gambacurta A. Blood derived stem cells: An

ameliorative therapy in veterinary ophthalmology. *J. Cell. Physiol.* 2012;227:1250–1256. doi: 10.1002/jcp.22953.

446. Saldinger L.K., Nelson S.G., Bellone R.R., Lassaline M., Mack M., Walker N.J., Borjesson D.L. Horses with equine recurrent uveitis have an activated CD4+ T-cell phenotype that can be modulated by mesenchymal stem cells in vitro. *Vet. Ophthalmol.* 2020;23:160–170. doi: 10.1111/vop.12704.
447. Villatoro A.J., Fernández V., Claros S., Rico-Llanos G.A., Becerra J., Andrades J.A. Use of Adipose-Derived Mesenchymal Stem Cells in Keratoconjunctivitis Sicca in a Canine Model. *BioMed Res. Int.* 2015;2015:527926. doi: 10.1155/2015/527926
448. Sgrignoli M.R., Silva D.A., Nascimento F.F., Sgrignoli D.A.M., Nai G.A., da Silva M.G., de Barros M.A., Bittencourt M.K.W., de Morais B.P., Dinallo H.R., et al. Reduction in the inflammatory markers CD4, IL-1, IL-6 and TNFα in dogs with keratoconjunctivitis sicca treated topically with mesenchymal stem cells. *Stem Cell Res.* 2019;39:101525. doi: 10.1016/j.scr.2019.101525.
449. Sukoyan MA, Vatolin SY, et al. Embryonic stem cells derived from morulae, inner cell mass, and blastocysts of mink: comparisons of their pluripotencies. Embryo Dev. 1993;36(2):148–58
450. Larijani B, Esfahani EN, Amini P, Nikbin B, Alimoghaddam K, Amiri S, Malekzadeh R, Yazdi NM, Ghodsi M, Dowlati Y, Sahraian MA, Ghavamzadeh A. Stem cell therapy in treatment of different diseases. Acta Medica Iranica. 2012:79–96 https://www.ncbi.nlm.nih.gov/pubmed/22359076.

451. Sullivan S, Stacey GN, Akazawa C, et al. Quality guidelines for clinical-grade human induced pluripotent stem cell lines. Regenerative Med. 2018; https://doi.org/10.2217/rme-2018-0095.

452. Amps K, Andrews PW, et al. Screening ethnically diverse human embryonic stem cells identifies a chromosome 20 minimal amplicon conferring growth advantage. Nat. Biotechnol. 2011;*29*(12):1121–44.

453. Amit M, Itskovitz-Eldor J. Atlas of human pluripotent stem cells: derivation and culturing. New York: Humana Press; 2012.

454. Ludwig TE, Bergendahl V, Levenstein ME, Yu J, Probasco MD, Thomson JA. Feeder-independent culture of human embryonic stem cells. Nat Methods. 2006;3:637–46.

455. Kang MI. Transitional CpG methylation between promoters and retroelements of tissue-specific genes during human mesenchymal cell differentiation. J. Cell Biochem. 2007;102:224–39.

456. Vaes B, Craeye D, Pinxteren J. Quality control during manufacture of a stem cell therapeutic. BioProcess Int. 2012;10:50–5.

457. Bloushtain-Qimron N. Epigenetic patterns of embryonic and adult stem cells. Cell Cycle. 2009;8:809–17.

458. Brindley DA. Peak serum: implications of serum supply for cell therapy manufacturing. Regenerative Medicine. 2012;7:809–17.

459. Solter D, Knowles BB. Immunosurgery of mouse blastocyst. Proc Natl Acad Sci U S A. 1975;72:5099–102.

460. Hoepfl G, Gassmann M, Desbaillets I. Differentiating embryonic stem cells into embryoid bodies. Methods Mole Biol. 2004;254:79–98 https://doi.org/10.1385/1-59259-741-6:079.

461. Lim WF, Inoue-Yokoo T, Tan KS, Lai MI, Sugiyama D. Hematopoietic cell differentiation from embryonic and induced pluripotent stem cells. Stem Cell Res Ther. 2013;4(3):71. https://doi.org/10.1186/scrt222.
462. Mohr JC, de Pablo JJ, Palecek SP. 3-D microwell culture of human embryonic stem cells. Biomaterials. 2006;27(36):6032–42. https://doi.org/10.1016/j.biomaterials.2006.07.012.
463. Doetschman TC, Eistetter H, Katz M, Schmidt W, Kemler R. The in vitro development of blastocyst-derived embryonic stem cell lines: formation of the visceral yolk sac, blood islands, and myocardium. J Embryol Exp Morphol. 1985;87:27–45.
464. Kurosawa HY. Methods for inducing embryoid body formation: in vitro differentiation system of embryonic stem cells. J Biosci Bioeng. 2007;103:389–98.
465. Heins N, Englund MC, Sjoblom C, Dahl U, Tonning A, Bergh C, Lindahl A, Hanson C, Semb H. Derivation, characterization, and differentiation of human embryonic stem cells. Stem Cells. 2004;22:367–76.
466. Rosowski KA, Mertz AF, Norcross S, Dufresne ER, Horsley V. Edges of human embryonic stem cell colonies display distinct mechanical properties and differentiation potential. Sci Rep. 2015;5:Article number:14218.
467. Chung Y, Klimanskaya I, Becker S, Li T, Maserati M, Lu SJ, Zdravkovic T, Ilic D, Genbacev O, Fisher S, Krtolica A, Lanza R. Human embryonic stem cell lines generated without embryo destruction. Cell Stem Cell. 2008;2:113–7.
468. Zhang X, Stojkovic P, Przyborski S, Cooke M, Armstrong L, Lako M, Stojkovic M. Derivation of human embryonic stem cells from developing and arrested embryos. Stem Cells. 2006;24:2669–76.

469. Beers J, Gulbranson DR, George N, Siniscalchi LI, Jones J, Thomson JA, Chen G. Passaging and colony expansion of human pluripotent stem cells by enzyme-free dissociation in chemically defined culture conditions. Nat Protoc. 2012;7:2029–40.

470. Ellerström C, Hyllner J, Strehl R. single cell enzymatic dissociation of human embryonic stem cells: a straightforward, robust, and standardized culture method. In: Turksen K, editor. Human embryonic stem cell protocols. Methods in molecular biology: Humana Press; 2009. p. 584.

471. Heng BC, Liu H, Ge Z, Cao T. Mechanical dissociation of human embryonic stem cell colonies by manual scraping after collagenase treatment is much more detrimental to cellular viability than is trypsinization with gentle pipetting. Biotechnol Appl Biochem. 2010;47(1):33–7.

472. Ellerstrom C, Strehl R, Noaksson K, Hyllner J, Semb H. Facilitated expansion of human embryonic stem cells by single-cell enzymatic dissociation. Stem Cells. 2007;25:1690–6.

473. Brimble SN, Zeng X, Weiler DA, Luo Y, Liu Y, Lyons IG, Freed WJ, Robins AJ, Rao MS, Schulz TC. Karyotypic stability, genotyping, differentiation, feeder-free maintenance, and gene expression sampling in three human embryonic stem cell lines deri. Stem Cells Dev. 2004;13:585–97.

474. Watanabe K, Ueno M, Kamiya D, Nishiyama A, Matsumura M, Wataya T, Takahashi JB, Nishikawa S, Nishikawa S, Muguruma K, Sasai Y. A ROCK inhibitor permits survival of dissociated human embryonic stem cells. Nat Biotechnol. 2007;25:681–6.

475. Nie Y, Walsh P, Clarke DL, Rowley JA, Fellner T. Scalable passaging of adherent human pluripotent stem cells. 2014. https://doi.org/10.1371/journal.pone.0088012.

476. Thomson JA, Itskovitz-Eldor J, Shapiro SS, Waknitz MA, Swiergiel JJ, Marshall VS, Jones JM. Embryonic stem cell lines derived from human blastocysts. Science. 1998;282:1145–7.
477. Martin MJ, Muotri A, Gage F, Varki A. Human embryonic stem cellsexpress an immunogenic nonhuman sialic acid. Nat. Med. 2005;11:228–32.
478. Smith AG, Heath JK, Donaldson DD, Wong GG, Moreau J, Stahl M, Rogers D. Inhibition of pluripotential embryonic stem cell differentiation by purified polypeptides. Nature. 1988;336(6200):688–90. https://doi.org/10.1038/336688a0.
479. Xu C, Inokuma MS, Denham J, Golds K, Kundu P, Gold JD, Carpenter MK. Feeder-free growth of undifferentiated human embryonic stem cells. Nature Biotechnol. 2001;19:971–4. https://doi.org/10.1038/nbt1001-971.
480. Weathersbee PS, Pool TB, Ord T. Synthetic serum substitute (SSS): a globulin-enriched protein supplement for human embryo culture. J. Assist Reprod Genet. 1995;12:354–60.
481. Chen G, Gulbranson DR, Hou Z, Bolin JM, Ruotti V, Probasco MD, Smuga-Otto K, Howden SE, Diol NR, Propson NE, Wagner R, Lee GO, Antosiewicz-Bourget J, Teng JM, Thomson JA. Chemically defined conditions for human iPSC derivation and culture. Nat. Methods. 2011;8:424–9.
482. Sommer CA, Mostoslavsky G. Experimental approaches for the generation of induced pluripotent stem cells. Stem Cell Res Ther. 2010;1:26.
483. Takahashi K, Yamanaka S. Induced pluripotent stem cells in medicine and biology. Development. 2013;140(12):2457–61 https://doi.org/10.1242/dev.092551.

484. Shi D, Lu F, Wei Y, et al. Buffalos (*Bubalus bubalis*) cloned by nuclear transfer of somatic cells. Biol. Reprod. 2007;77:285–91. https://doi.org/10.1095/biolreprod.107.060210.

485. Gurdon JB. The developmental capacity of nuclei taken from intestinal epithelium cells of feeding tadpoles. Development. 1962;10:622–40 http://dev.biologists.org/content/10/4/622.

486. Kain K. The birth of cloning: an interview with John Gurdon. Dis Model Mech. 2009;2(1–2):9–10. https://doi.org/10.1242/dmm.002014.

487. Davis RL, Weintraub H, Lassar AB. Expression of a single transfected cDNA converts fibroblasts to myoblasts. Cell. 1987;24(51(6)):987–1000.

488. Quinlan AR, Boland MJ, Leibowitz ML, et al. Genome sequencing of mouse induced pluripotent stem cells reveals retroelement stability and infrequent DNA rearrangement during reprogramming. Cell Stem Cell. 2011;9(4):366–73.

489. Maherali N, Sridharan R, Xie W, Utika LJ, Eminli S, Arnold K, Stadtfeld M, Yachechko R, Tchieu J, Jaenisch R, Plath K, Hochedlinger K. Directly reprogrammed fibroblasts show global epigenetic remodeling and widespread tissue contribution. Cell Stem Cell. 2007;1:55–70.

490. Ohi Y, Qin H, Hong C, Blouin L, Polo JM, Guo T, Qi Z, Downey SL, Manos PD, Rossi DJ, Yu J, Hebrok M, Hochedlinger K, Costello JF, Song JS, Ramalho-Santos M. Incomplete DNA methylation underlines a transcriptional memory of somatic cells in human IPS cells. Nat Cell Biol. 2011;13:541–9.

491. Zhou Q, Brown J, Kanarek A, Rajagopal J, Melton DA. In vivo reprogramming of adult pancreatic exocrine cells to beta-cells. Nature. 2008;455:627–32 https://doi.org/10.1038/nature07314.

492. Hilfiker A, Kasper C, Hass R, Haverich A. Mesenchymal stem cells and progenitor cells in connective tissue engineering and regenerative medicine: is there a future for transplantation? Langenbecks Arch Surg. 2011;396:489–97.
493. Zhang Wendy, Y., de Almeida Patricia, E., and Wu Joseph, C. Teratoma formation: a tool for monitoring pluripotency in stem cell research. StemBook, ed. The Stem Cell Research Community. June 12, 2012. https://doi.org/10.3824/stembook.1.53.1.
494. Narsinh KH, Sun N, Sanchez-Freire V, et al. Single cell transcriptional profiling reveals heterogeneity of human induced pluripotent stem cells. J Clin Invest. 2011;121(3):1217–21.
495. Gertow K, Przyborski S, Loring JF, Auerbach JM, Epifano O, Otonkoski T, Damjanov I, AhrlundRichter L. Isolation of human embryonic stem cell-derived teratomas for the assessment of pluripotency. Curr Protoc Stem Cell Biol. 2007, Chapter 1, Unit 1B 4. 3: 1B.4.1-1B.4.29.
496. Cooke MJ, Stojkovic M, Przyborski SA. Growth of teratomas derived from human pluripotent stem cells is influenced by the graft site. Stem Cells Dev. 2006;15(2):254–9.
497. Przyborski SA. Differentiation of human embryonic stem cells after transplantation in immune-deficient mice. Stem Cells. 2005;23:1242–50.
498. Tannenbaum SE, Turetsky TT, Singer O, Aizenman E, Kirshberg S, Ilouz N, Gil Y, Berman-Zaken Y, Perlman TS, Geva N, Levy O, Arbell D, Simon A, Ben-Meir A, Shufaro Y, Laufer N, Reubinoff BE. Derivation of xeno-free and GMP-grade human embryonic stem cells- platforms for future clinical applications. PLoS One. 2012;7:e35325.
499. Cohen DE, Melton D. Turning straw into gold: directing cell fate for regenerative medicine. Nat Rev Genet. 2011;12:243–52.

500. Hwang NS, Varghese S, Elisseeff J. Controlled differentiation of stem cells. Adv Drug Deliv Rev. 2007;60(2):199–214. https://doi.org/10.1016/j.addr.2007.08.036.
501. Turner N, Grose R. Fibroblast growth factor signalling: from development to cancer. Nat Rev Cancer. 2010;10:116–29.
502. Rao TP, Kuhl M. An updated overview on Wnt signaling pathways: a prelude for more. Circ Res. 2010;106:1798–806.
503. Moustakas A, Heldin CH. The regulation of TGFbeta signal transduction. Development. 2009;136:3699–714.
504. Efthymiou AG, Chen G, Rao M, Chen G, Boehm M. Self-renewal and cell lineage differentiation strategies in human embryonic stem cells and induced pluripotent stem cells. Expert Opin Biol Ther. 2014;14:1333–44.
505. Yang L, Soonpaa MH, Adler ED, Roepke TK, Kattman SJ, Kennedy M, Henckaerts E, Bonham K, Abbott GW, Linden RM, Field LJ, Keller GM. Human cardiovascular progenitor cells develop from a KDRþembryonic-stem-cell-derived population. Nature. 2008;453:524–8.
506. Kroon E, Martinson LA, Kadoya K, Bang AG, Kelly OG, Eliazer S, Young H, Richardson M, Smart NG, Cunningham J, Agulnick AD, D'amour KA, Carpenter MK, Baetge EE. Pancreatic endoderm derived from human embryonic stem cells generates glucose-responsive insulin-secreting cells in vivo. Nat Biotechnol. 2008;26(4):443–52. https://doi.org/10.1038/nbt1393.
507. Vallier L, Reynolds D, Pedersen RA. Nodal inhibits differentiation of human embryonic stem cells along the neuroectodermal default pathway. Dev Biol. 2004;275:403–21.

508. Burridge PW, Zambidis ET. Highly efficient directed differentiation of human induced pluripotent stem cells into cardiomyocytes. Methods Mol Biol. 2013;997:149–61.
509. Cai J, Zhao Y, Liu Y, Ye F, Song Z, Qin H, Meng S, Chen Y, Zhou R, Song X, Guo Y, Ding M, Deng H. Directed differentiation of human embryonic stem cells into functional hepatic cells. Hepatology. 2007;45:1229–39.
510. Takasato M, Er PX, Becroft M, Vanslambrouck JM, Stanley EG, Elefanty AG, Little MH. Directing human embryonic stem cell differentiation towards a renal lineage generates a selforganizing kidney. Nat Cell Biol. 2014;16:118–26.
511. Huang SX, Islam MN, O'Neill J, Hu Z, Yang YG, Chen YW, Mumau M, Green MD, VunjakNovakovic G, Bhattacharya J, Snoeck HW. Efficient generation of lung and airway epithelial cells from human pluripotent stem cells. Nat Biotechnol. 2014;32:84–91.
512. Kadzik RS, Morrisey EE. Directing lung endoderm differentiation in pluripotent stem cells. Cell Stem Cell. 2012;10:355–61.
513. Wichterle H, Lieberam I, Porter JA, Jessell TM. Directed differentiation of embryonic stem cells into motor neurons. Cell. 2002;110:385–97.
514. Spence JR, Mayhew CN, Rankin SA, Kuhar MF, Vallance JE, Tolle K, Hoskins EE, Kalinichenko VV, Wells SI, Zorn AM, Shroyer NF, Wells JM. Directed differentiation of human pluripotent stem cells into intestinal tissue in vitro. Nature. 2011;470:105–9.
515. Oldershaw RA, Baxter MA, Lowe ET, Bates N, Grady LM, Soncin F, Brison DR, Hardingham TE, Kimber SJ. Directed differentiation of human embryonic stem cells toward chondrocytes. Nat Biotechnol. 2010;28:1187–94.

516. Jun Cai, Ann DeLaForest, Joseph Fisher, Amanda Urick, Thomas Wagner, Kirk Twaroski, Max Cayo, Masato Nagaoka, Stephen A Duncan. Protocol for directed differentiation of human pluripotent stem cells toward a hepatocyte fate. 2012. DOI: https://doi.org/10.3824/stembook.1.52.1.

517. Frank-Kamenetsky M, Zhang XM, Bottega S, Guicherit O, Wichterle H, Dudek H, Bumcrot D, Wang FY, Jones S, Shulok J, Rubin LL, Porter JA. Small-molecule modulators of hedgehog signaling: identification and characterization of smoothened agonists and antagonists. J Biol. 2002;1:10.

518. Oshima K, Shin K, Diensthuber M, Peng AW, Ricci AJ, Heller S. Mechanosensitive hair celllike cells from embryonic and induced pluripotent stem cells. Cell. 2010;141:704–16.

519. Osakada F, Jin ZB, Hirami Y, Ikeda H, Danjyo T, Watanabe K, Sasai Y, Takahashi M. In vitro differentiation of retinal cells from human pluripotent stem cells by small-molecule induction. J Cell Sci. 2009;122:3169–79.

520. Kshitiz PJ, Kim P, Helen W, Engler AJ, Levchenko A, Kim DH. Control of stem cell fate and function by engineering physical microenvironments. Intergr Biol (Camb). 2012;4:1008–18.

521. Amps K, Andrews PW, Anyfantis G, Armstrong L, Avery S, Baharvand H, Baker J, Baker D, Munoz MB, Beil S, Benvenisty N, Ben-Yosef D, Biancotti JC, Bosman A, Brena RM, Brison D, Caisander G, Camarasa MV, Chen J, ChiaoE CYM, Choo AB, Collins D, et al. Screening ethnically diverse human embryonic stem cells identifies a chromosome 20 minimal amplicon conferring growth advantage. Nat Biotechnol. 2011;29:1132–44.

522. Nukaya D, Minami K, Hoshikawa R, Yokoi N, Seino S. Preferential gene expression and epigenetic memory of induced pluripotent stem cells derived from mouse pancreas. Genes Cells. 2015;20:367–81.

523. Murdoch A, Braude P, Courtney A, Brison D, Hunt C, Lawford-Davies J, Moore H, Stacey G, Sethe S, Procurement Working Group Of National Clinical H, E. S. C. F, National Clinical H, E. S. C. F. The procurement of cells for the derivation of human embryonic stem cell lines for therapeutic use: recommendations for good practice. Stem Cell Rev. 2012;8:91–9.
524. Hewitson H, Wood V, Kadeva N, Cornwell G, Codognotto S, Stephenson E, Ilic D. Generation of KCL035 research grade human embryonic stem cell line carrying a mutation in HBB gene. Stem Cell Res. 2016;16:210–2.
525. Daley GQ, Hyun I, Apperley JF, Barker RA, Benvenisty N, Bredenoord AL, Breuer CK, Caulfield T, Cedars MI, Frey-Vasconcells J, Heslop HE, Jin Y, Lee RT, Mccabe C, Munsie M, Murry CE, Piantadosi S, Rao M, Rooke HM, Sipp D, Studer L, Sugarman J, et al. Setting global standards for stem cell research and clinical translation: the 2016 ISSCR guidelines. Stem Cell Rep. 2016;6:787–97.
526. Takahashi K, Yamanaka S. Induction of pluripotent stem cells from mouse embryonic and adult fibroblast cultures by defined factors. Cell. 2006;126(4):663–76. https://doi.org/10.1016/j.cell.2006.07.024.
527. Loh YH, Wu Q, Chew JL, Vega VB, Zhang W, Chen X, Bourque G, George J, Leong B, Liu J, et al. The Oct4 and Nanog transcription network regulates pluripotency in mouse embryonic stem cells. Nat Genet. 2006;38:431–40.
528. Menasche P, Vanneaux V, Hagege A, Bel A, Cholley B, Cacciapuoti I, Parouchev A, Benhamouda N, Tachdjian G, Tosca L, Trouvin JH, Fabreguettes JR, Bellamy V, Guillemain R, SuberbielleBoissel C, Tartour E, Desnos M, Larghero J. Human embryonic stem cell-derived cardiac progenitors for severe heart failure treatment: first clinical case report. Eur Heart J. 2015;36:2011–7.

529. Schwartz SD, Regillo CD, Lam BL, Eliott D, Rosenfeld PJ, Gregori NZ, Hubschman JP, Davis JL, Heilwell G, Spirn M, Maguire J, Gay R, Bateman J, Ostrick RM, Morris D, Vincent M, Anglade E, Del Priore LV, Lanza R. Human embryonic stem cell-derived retinal pigment epithelium in patients with age-related macular degeneration and Stargardt's macular dystrophy: follow-up of two open-label phase 1/2 studies. Lancet. 2015;385:509–16.
530. Ilic D, Ogilvie C. Concise review: human embryonic stem cells-what have we done? What are we doing? Where are we going? Stem Cells. 2017;35:17–25.
531. Rocha V, et al. Clinical use of umbilical cord blood hematopoietic stem cells. Biol Blood Marrow Transplant. 2006;12(1):34–4.
532. Longo UG, Ronga M, Maffulli N. Sports Med Arthrosc 17:112–126. Achilles tendinopathy. Sports Med Arthrosc. 2009;17:112–26.
533. Tempfer H, Lehner C, Grütz M, Gehwolf R, Traweger A. Biological augmentation for tendon repair: lessons to be learned from development, disease, and tendon stem cell research. In: Gimble J, Marolt D, Oreffo R, Redl H, Wolbank S, editors. Cell engineering and regeneration. Reference Series in Biomedical Engineering. Cham: Springer; 2017.
534. Goldring MB, Goldring SR. Osteoarthritis. J Cell Physiol. 2007;213:626–34.
535. Widuchowski W, Widuchowski J, Trzaska T. Articular cartilage defects: study of 25,124 knee arthroscopies. Knee. 2007;14:177–82.
536. Li R, Lin Q-X, Liang X-Z, Liu G-B, et al. Stem cell therapy for treating osteonecrosis of the femoral head: from clinical applications to related basic research. Stem Cell Res Therapy. 2018;9:291 https://doi.org/10.1186/s13287-018-1018-7.
537. Gangji V, De Maertelaer V, Hauzeur JP. Autologous bone marrow cell implantation in the treatment of non-traumatic osteonecrosis of the femoral

head: five year follow-up of a prospective controlled study. Bone. 2011;49(5):1005–9.

538. Zhao D, Cui D, Wang B, Tian F, Guo L, Yang L, et al. Treatment of early stage osteonecrosis of the femoral head with autologous implantation of bone marrow-derived and cultured mesenchymal stem cells. Bone. 2012;50(1):325–30.

539. Sen RK, Tripathy SK, Aggarwal S, Marwaha N, Sharma RR, Khandelwal N. Early results of core decompression and autologous bone marrow mononuclear cells instillation in femoral head osteonecrosis: a randomized control study. J Arthroplast. 2012;27(5):679–86.

540. Lapasset L, Milhavet O, Prieur A, Besnard E, Babled A, Aït-Hamou N, Leschik J, Pellestor F, Ramirez JM, De Vos J, Lehmann S, Lemaitre JM. Rejuvenating senescent and centenarian human cells by reprogramming through the pluripotent state. Genes Dev. 2011;25:2248–53.

541. Sahin E, Depinho RA. Linking functional decline of telomeres, mitochondria and stem cells during ageing. Nature. 2010;464:520–8.

542. Petkovich DA, Podolskiy DI, Lobanov AV, Lee SG, Miller RA, Gladyshev VN. Using DNA methylation profiling to evaluate biological age and longevity interventions. Cell Metab. 2017;25:954–60 https://doi.org/10.1016/j.cmet.2017.03.016.

543. Gerontology, Rejuvenation by cell reprogramming: a new horizon in. Rodolfo G. Goya, Marianne Lehmann, Priscila Chiavellini, Martina Canatelli-Mallat, Claudia B. Hereñú and Oscar A. Brown. Stem Cell Res Therapy. 2018, 9:349. https://doi.org/10.1186/s13287-018-1075-y.

544. Ocampo A, Reddy P, Martinez-Redondo P, Platero-Luengo A, Hatanaka F, Hishida T, Li M, Lam D, Kurita M, Beyret E, Araoka T, Vazquez-Ferrer E,

Donoso D, Roman JLXJ, Rodriguez-Esteban C, Nuñez G, Nuñez Delicado E, Campistol JM, Guillen I, Guillen P, Izpisua. In vivo amelioration of age-associated hallmarks by partial reprogramming. Cell. 2016;167:1719–33.

545. de Lázaro I, Cossu G, Kostarelos K. Transient transcription factor (OSKM) expression is key towards clinical translation of in vivo cell reprogramming. EMBO Mol Med. 2017;9:733–6.

546. Sun S, Li ZQ, Glencer P, Cai BC, Zhang XM, Yang J, Li XR. Bringing the age-related macular degeneration high-risk allele age-related maculopathy susceptibility 2 into focus with stem cell technology. Stem Cell Res Ther. 2017;8:135 https://doi.org/10.1186/s13287-017-0584-4.

547. Liu J. Induced pluripotent stem cell-derived neural stem cells: new hope for stroke? Stem Cell Res Ther. 2013;4:115 https://doi.org/10.1186/scrt326.

548. Shahjalal HM, Dayem AA, Lim KM, Jeon TI, Cho SG. Generation of pancreatic β cells for treatment of diabetes: advances and challenges. Stem Cell ResTher. 2018;9:355 https://doi.org/10.1186/s13287-018-1099-3.

549. Kroon E, Martinson LA, et al. Pancreatic endoderm derived from human embryonic stem cells generates glucose-responsive insulin-secreting cells in vivo. Nat Biotechnol. 2008;26;443–52.

550. Arora V, Pooja A, Munshi AK. Banking stem cells from human exfoliated deciduous teeth. J Clin Pediatr Dent. 2009;33(4):289–94.

551. Mao JJ. Stem cells and the future of dental care. New York State Dental J. 2008;74(2):21–4.

552. Reznick, Jay B. Continuing education: stem cells: emerging medical and dental therapies for the dental Professional. Dentaltown Magazine. 2008, pp. 42–53.

553. Arthur A, Rychkov G, Shi S, Koblar SA, Gronthos S. Adult human dental pulp stem cells differentiate toward functionally active neurons under appropriate environmental cues. Stem Cells. 2008;26(7):1787–95.
554. Cordeiro MM, Dong Z, Kaneko T, Zhang Z, Miyazawa M, Shi S, Smith A. Dental pulp tissue engineering with stem cells from exfoliated. J Endod. 2008;34(8):962–9.
555. Hayashi K, Ohta H, Kurimoto K, Aramaki S, Saitou M. Reconstitution of the mouse germ cell specification pathway in culture by pluripotent stem cells. Cell. 2011;146(4):519–32. https://doi.org/10.1016/j.cell.2011.06.052.
556. Sadri-Ardekani H, Atala A. Testicular tissue cryopreservation and spermatogonial stem cell transplantation to restore fertility: from bench to bedside. Stem Cell ResTher. 2014;5:68 https://doi.org/10.1186/scrt457.
557. Zhang Q, Xu M, Yao X, Li T, Wang Q, Lai D. Human amniotic epithelial cells inhibit granulosa cell apoptosis induced by chemotherapy and restore the fertility. Stem Cell Res Ther. 2015;6:152 https://doi.org/10.1186/s13287-015-0148-4.
558. Ma DK, Bonaguidi MA, Ming GL, Song H. Adult neural stem cells in the mammalian central nervous system. Cell Res. 2009;19:672–82. https://doi.org/10.1038/cr.2009.56.
559. Dantuma E, Merchant S, Sugaya K. Stem cells for the treatment of neurodegenerative diseases. Stem Cell ResTher. 2010;1:37 https://doi.org/10.1186/scrt37.
560. Wang Q, Matsumoto Y, Shindo T, Miyake K, Shindo A, Kawanishi M, Kawai N, Tamiya T, Nagao S. Neural stem cells transplantation in cortex in a mouse model of Alzheimer's disease. J Med Invest. 2006;53:61–9. https://doi.org/10.2152/jmi.53.61.

561. Moghadam FH, Alaie H, Karbalaie K, Tanhaei S, Nasr Esfahani MH, Baharvand H. Transplantation of primed or unprimed mouse embryonic stem cell-derived neural precursor cells improves cognitive function in Alzheimerian rats. Differentiation. 2009;78:59–68. https://doi.org/10.1016/j.diff.2009.06.005.
562. Byrne JA. Developing neural stem cell-based treatments for neurodegenerative diseases. Stem Cell ResTher. 2014;5:72. https://doi.org/10.1186/scrt461.
563. Awe JP, Lee PC, Ramathal C, Vega-Crespo A, Durruthy-Durruthy J, Cooper A, Karumbayaram S, Lowry WE, Clark AT, Zack JA, Sebastiano V, Kohn DB, Pyle AD, Martin MG, Lipshutz GS, Phelps PE, Pera RA, Byrne JA. Generation and characterization of transgene-free human induced pluripotent stem cells and conversion to putative clinical-grade status. Stem Cell Res Ther. 2013;4:87. https://doi.org/10.1186/scrt246.
564. Peng J, Zeng X. The role of induced pluripotent stem cells in regenerative medicine: neurodegenerative diseases. Stem Cell ResTher. 2011;2:32. https://doi.org/10.1186/scrt73.
565. Wright BL, Barker RA. Established and emerging therapies for Huntington's disease. 2007;7(6):579–87 https://www.ncbi.nlm.nih.gov/pubmed/17896994/579-87.
566. Lin NH, Gronthos S, Bartold PM. Stem cells and periodontal regeneration. Aust Dent J. 2008;53:108–21.
567. Seo BM, Miura M, Gronthos S, Bartold PM, Batouli S, Brahim J, et al. Investigation of multipotent postnatal stem cells from human periodontal ligament. Lancet. 2004;364:149–55.

568. Ramseier CA, Abramson ZR, Jin Q, Giannobile WV. Gene therapeutics for periodontal regenerative medicine. Dent Clin North Am. 2006;50:245–63.
569. Shi S, Bartold PM, Miura M, Seo BM, Robey PG, Gronthos S. The efficacy of mesenchymal stem cells to regenerate and repair dental structures. OrthodCraniofac Res. 2005;8:191–9.
570. Iohara K, Nakashima M, Ito M, Ishikawa M, Nakasima A, Akamine A. Dentin regeneration by dental pulp stem cell therapy with recombinant human bone morphogenetic protein. J Dent Res. 2004;83:590–5.
571. Hu B, Unda F, Bopp-Kuchler S, Jimenez L, Wang XJ, Haikel Y, et al. Bone marrow cells can give rise to ameloblast-like cells. J Dent Res. 2006;85:416–21.
572. Liu Y, Liu W, Hu C, Xue Z, Wang G, Ding B, Luo H, Tang L, Kong X, Chen X, Liu N, Ding Y, Jin Y. MiR-17 modulates osteogenic differentiation through a coherent feed-forward loop in mesenchymal stem cells isolated from periodontal ligaments of patients with periodontitis. Stem Cells. 2011;29(11):1804–16. https://doi.org/10.1002/stem.728.
573. Raspini G, Wolff J, Helminen M, Raspini G, Raspini M, Sándor GK. Dental stem cells harvested from third molars combined with bioactive glass can induce signs of bone formation in vitro. J Oral Maxillofac Res. 2018;9(1):e2. Published 2018 Mar 31. https://doi.org/10.5037/jomr.2018.9102.
574. Christodoulou I, Goulielmaki M, Devetzi M, Panagiotidis M, Koliakos G, Zoumpourlis V. Mesenchymal stem cells in preclinical cancer cytotherapy: a systematic review. Stem Cell Res Ther. 2018;9(1;336). https://doi.org/10.1186/s13287-018-1078-8.

575. Bansal R, Jain A. Current overview on dental stem cells applications in regenerative dentistry. J Nat Sci Biol Med. 2015;6(1):29–34. https://doi.org/10.4103/0976-9668.149074.
576. Edgar Ledesma-Martínez, Víctor Manuel Mendoza-Núñez, Edelmiro Santiago-Osorio. Mesenchymal stem cells derived from dental pulp: a review. Stem Cells Int. 2016, 4,709,572, p. doi: https://doi.org/10.1155/2016/4709572].
577. Grzech-Leśniak K. Making use of lasers in periodontal treatment: a new gold standard? Photomed Laser Surg. 2017;35(10):513–4.
578. Miura M, Gronthos S, Zhao M, Lu B, Fisher LW, Robey PG, Shi S. SHED: stem cells from human exfoliated deciduous teeth. Proc Natl Acad Sci U S A. 2003;100(10):5807–12. https://doi.org/10.1073/pnas.0937635100.
579. Yasui T, Mabuchi Y, Toriumi H, Ebine T, Niibe K, Houlihan DD, Morikawa S, Onizawa K, Kawana H, Akazawa C, Suzuki N, Nakagawa T, Okano H, Matsuzaki Y. Purified human dental pulp stem cells promote osteogenic regeneration. J Dent Res. 2016;95(2):206–14. https://doi.org/10.1177/0022034515610748.
580. Yamamoto A, Sakai K, Matsubara K, Kano F, Ueda M. Multifaceted neuro-regenerative activities of human dental pulp stem cells for functional recovery after spinal cord injury. Neurosci Res. 2014;78:16–20. https://doi.org/10.1016/j.neures.2013.10.010.
581. d'Aquino R, De Rosa A, Lanza V, Tirino V, Laino L, Graziano A, Desiderio V, Laino G, Papaccio G. Human mandible bone defect repair by the grafting of dental pulp stem/progenitor cells and collagen sponge biocomplexes. Eur Cell Mater. 2009;12, PMID: 19908196:75–83.

582. Wang L, Shen H, Zheng W, Tang L, Yang Z, Gao Y, Yang Q, Wang C, Duan Y, Jin Y. Characterization of stem cells from alveolar periodontal ligament. Tissue Eng. Part A. 2011;17(7–8):1015–26. https://doi.org/10.1089/ten.tea.2010.0140.
583. Iwata T, Yamato M, Zhang Z, Mukobata S, Washio K, Ando T, Feijen J, Okano T, Ishikawa I. Validation of human periodontal ligament-derived cells as a reliable source for cytotherapeutic use. J Clin Periodontol. 2010;37(12):1088–99. https://doi.org/10.1111/j.1600-051X.2010.01597.x.
584. Chen F-M, Gao L-N, Tian B-M, Zhang X-Y, Zhang Y-J, Dong G-Y, Lu H, et al. Treatment of periodontal intrabony defects using autologous periodontal ligament stem cells: a randomized clinical trial. Stem Cell Res Ther. 2016;7:33. https://doi.org/10.1186/s13287-016-0288-1.
585. Bakopoulou A, Leyhausen G, Volk J, Tsiftsoglou A, Garefis P, Koidis P, Geurtsen W. Comparative analysis of in vitro osteo/odontogenic differentiation potential of human dental pulp stem cells (DPSCs) and stem cells from the apical papilla (SCAP). Arch Oral Biol. 2011;56(7):709–21. https://doi.org/10.1016/j.archoralbio.2010.12.008.
586. Han C, Yang Z, Zhou W, Jin F, Song Y, Wang Y, Huo N, Chen L, Qian H, Hou R, Duan Y, Jin Y. Periapical follicle stem cell: a promising candidate for cementum/periodontal ligament regeneration and bio-root engineering. Stem Cells Dev. 2010;19(9):1405–15. https://doi.org/10.1089/scd.2009.0277.
587. Luan X, Ito Y, Dangaria S, Diekwisch TG. Dental follicle progenitor cell heterogeneity in the developing mouse periodontium. Stem Cells Dev. 2006;15(4):595–608. https://doi.org/10.1089/scd.2006.15.595.
588. Handa K, Saito M, Tsunoda A, Yamauchi M, Hattori S, Sato S, Toyoda M, Teranaka T, Narayanan AS. Progenitor cells from dental follicle are able to

form cementum matrix in vivo. Connect Tissue Res. 2002;43(2–3):406–8 PMID: 12489190.

589. Guo W, Chen L, Gong K, Ding B, Duan Y, Jin Y. Heterogeneous dental follicle cells and the regeneration of complex periodontal tissues. Tissue Engineering. Part A. 2012;18(5–6):459–70 https://doi.org/10.1089/ten.tea.2011.0261.
590. Bai, Yudi et al. Cementum- and periodontal ligament-like tissue formation by dental follicle cell sheets co-cultured with Hertwig's epithelial root sheath cells. Bone. 2011, 48, Issue 6, pp. 1417–1426, https://doi.org/10.1016/j.bone.2011.02.016.
591. Cordeiro MM, Dong Z, Kaneko T, Zhang Z, Miyazawa M, Shi S, et al. Dental pulp tissue engineering with stem cells from exfoliated deciduous teeth. 2008, 34, pp. 962–969.
592. Dobie K, Smith G, Sloan AJ, Smith AJ. Effects of alginate, hydrogels and TGF-beta 1 on human dental pulp repair in vitro. Connect Tissue Res 2. 2002;43:387–90.
593. Friedlander LT, Cullinan MP, Love RM. Dental stem cells and their potential role in apexogenesis and apexification. Int Endod J. 2009;42:955–62.
594. Cai J, Zhang Y, Liu P, Chen S, Wu X, Sun Y, Li A, Huang K, Luo R, Wang L, Liu Y, Zhou T, Wei S, Pan G, Pei D, Generation of tooth-like structures from integration-free human urine induced pluripotent stem cells. Cell Regen (Lond). July 30, 2013, 2(1), pp. 6, doi: https://doi.org/10.1186/2045-9769-2-6.
595. Craig J. Taylor, Eleanor M. Bolton, and J. Andrew Bradley 2011 Aug 12 and https://doi.org/10.1098/rstb.2011.0030], 366(1575): 2312–2322. [doi:. Immunological considerations for embryonic and induced pluripotent stem

cell banking,. Philos Trans R SocLond B Biol Sci. 2011, 366(1575), pp. 2312–2322, doi:https://doi.org/10.1098/rstb.2011.0030.

596. T.R. Nayak, H. Andersen, V.S. Makam, C. Khaw, S. Bae, X.F. Xu, P.L.R. Ee, J.H. Ahn, B.H. Hong, G. Pastorin, B. Ozyilmaz, ACS Nano, 5 (6) (2011), pp. 4. Graphene for controlled and accelerated osteogenic differentiation of human mesenchymal stem cells,. ACS Nano. 2011, pp. 4670–4678.
597. Lee WC, Lim C, Shi H, Tang LAL, Wang Y, Lim CT, Loh KP. Origin of enhanced stem cell growth and differentiation on graphene and graphene oxide. ACS Nano. 2011;5(9):7334–41.
598. Kenry LWC, Loh KP, Lim CT. When stem cells meet graphene: opportunities and challenges in regenerative medicine. Biomaterials. 2018;155:236–50.
599. Yuan A, Farber EL, Rapoport AL, Tejada D, Deniskin R, Akhmedov NB, et al. Transfer of microRNAs by embryonic stem cell microvesicles. 2009. 2009, 4(3), p. https://doi.org/10.1371/journal.pone. 0004722.
600. Oh, Myeongsik, et al. Exosomes derived from human induced pluripotent stem cells ameliorate the aging of skin fibroblasts. Int. J. Mol. Sci. 2018, 19(6), p. 1715.
601. Ramirez MI. et al. Technical challenges of working with extracellular vesicles. Nanoscale. 2018;10:881–906.
602. Valadi H, et al. Exosome-mediated transfer of mRNAs and microRNAs is a novel mechanism of genetic exchange between cells. Nat. Cell Biol. 2007;9:654–9.
603. Mateescu B, et al. Obstacles and opportunities in the functional analysis of extracellular vesicle RNA—an ISEV position paper. J. Extracell. Vesicles. 2017;6(1). https://doi.org/10.1080/20013078.2017.1286095.

604. Nawaz M, et al. Extracellular vesicles: evolving factors in stem cell biology. Stem Cells Int. 2016;2016:17. Article ID 1073140.
605. Helfrich, Y.R., Sachs, D.L. and Voorhees, J.J. Overview of skin aging and photoaging. Dermatol. Nurs. 20, pp. 177–183, https://www.ncbi.nlm.nih.gov/pubmed/18649702.
606. Julia Tigges, Jean Krutmann, Ellen Fritsche, Judith Haendeler, Heiner Schaal, Jens W. Fischer, Faiza Kalfalah, Hans Reinke, Guido Reifenberger, Kai Stühler, Natascia Ventura, Sabrina Gundermann, Petra Boukamp, Fritz Boege. The hallmarks of fibroblast ageing, mechanisms of ageing and development, 138, 2014, Pages 26–44. 2014, 138, pp. 26–44, ISSN 0047–6374, https://doi.org/10.1016/j.mad.2014.03.004.
607. Huh MI, Kim MS, Kim HK, et al. Effect of conditioned media collected from human amniotic fluid-derived stem cells (hAFSCs) on skin regeneration and photo-aging. Tissue Eng Regen Med. 2014;11:171 https://doi.org/10.1007/s13770-014-0412-1.
608. Togel F, Hu Z, Weiss K, et al. Administered mesenchymal stem cells protect against ischemic acute renal failure through differentiation-independent mechanisms. Am J Physiol Renal Physiol. 2005;289:F31.
609. Liu J, Han G, Liu H, et al. Suppression of cholangiocarcinoma cell growth by human umbilical cord mesenchymal stem cells: a possible role of Wnt and Akt signaling. PLoS One. 2013;8:e62844.
610. Oh M, et al. Promotive effects of human induced pluripotent stem cell-conditioned medium on the proliferation and migration of dermal fibroblasts. Biotechnol. Bioprocess Eng. 2017;22:561–8.

611. Chen L, Tredget EE, Wu PY, Wu Y. Paracrine factors of mesenchymal stem cells recruit macrophages and endothelial lineage cells and enhance wound healing. PloS One. 2008;3:e1886.

612. Bae J-S, Lee S-H, Kim J-E, Choi J-Y, Park R-W, Park JY, Park H-S, Sohn Y-S, Lee D-S, Lee EB. βig-h3 supports keratinocyte adhesion, migration, and proliferation through α3β1 integrin. Biochem. Biophys. Res. Commun. 2002;294:940–8.

613. Zhou B-R, Xu Y, Guo S-L, Xu Y, Wang Y, Zhu F, Permatasari F, Wu D, Yin Z-Q, Luo D. The effect of conditioned media of adipose-derived stem cells on wound healing after ablative fractional carbon dioxide laser resurfacing. BioMed Res. Int. 2013;519:126.

614. Peng Y, Baulier E, Ke Y, Young A, Ahmedli NB, Schwartz SD, et al. Human embryonic stem cells extracellular vesicles and their effects on immortalized human retinal Müller cells. PLoS ONE. 2018, 13(3), p. https://doi.org/10.1371/journal.pone.019400.

615. Harris MT, Butler DL, Boivin GP, Florer JB, Schantz EJ, Wenstrup RJ. Mesenchymal stem cells used for rabbit tendon repair can form ectopic bone and express alkaline phosphatase activity in constructs. J Orthop Res. 2004;22:998–1003.

616. Mascetti VL, Pedersen RA. Human-mouse chimerism validates human stem cell pluripotency. Cell Stem Cell. 2016;18:67–72.

617. Curry, S.H. Translational Science: Past, Present, and Future. *BioTechniques* **2008**, *44*, ii–viii. [

618. Carbone, L. Pain in Laboratory Animals: The Ethical and Regulatory Imperatives. *PLoS ONE* **2011**, *6*, e21578.

619. Pritt, S.L.; Hammer, R.E. The Interplay of Ethics, Animal Welfare, and IACUC Oversight on the Reproducibility of Animal Studies. *Comp. Med.* **2017**, *67*, 101–105.

620. Frasch, P.D. Gaps in US Animal Welfare Law for Laboratory Animals: Perspectives From an Animal Law Attorney. *ILAR J.* **2016**, *57*, 285–292.

621. Hubrecht, R.C.; Carter, E. The 3Rs and Humane Experimental Technique: Implementing Change. *Animals* **2019**, *9*, 754

622. Seyhan, A.A. Lost in Translation: The Valley of Death across Preclinical and Clinical Divide–Identification of Problems and Overcoming Obstacles. *Transl. Med. Commun.* **2019**, *4*, 18.

623. Hickman, D.L.; Johnson, J.; Vemulapalli, T.H.; Crisler, J.R.; Shepherd, R. Commonly Used Animal Models. In *Principles of Animal Research for Graduate and Undergraduate Students*; Academic Press: Cambridge, MA, USA, 2017; pp. 117–175.

624. Perlman, R.L. Mouse Models of Human Disease: An Evolutionary Perspective. *Evol. Med. Public Health* **2016**, *2016*, 170–176.

625. Farrell, G.; Schattenberg, J.M.; Leclercq, I.; Yeh, M.M.; Goldin, R.; Teoh, N.; Schuppan, D. Mouse Models of Nonalcoholic Steatohepatitis: Toward Optimization of Their Relevance to Human Nonalcoholic Steatohepatitis. *Hepatology* **2019**, *69*, 2241–2257.

626. Oligschlaeger, Y.; Shiri-Sverdlov, R. NAFLD Preclinical Models: More than a Handful, Less of a Concern? *Biomedicines* **2020**, *8*, 28.

627. Cook, R.; Karesh, W.; Osofsky, S. *One World, One Health: Building Interdisciplinary Bridges to Health in a Globalized World*; Wildlife Conservation Society: Bronx, NY, USA, 2004; Available

online: **https://www.oneworldonehealth.org/sept2004/owohsept04.html** (accessed on 18 April 2016).

628. Evans, B.R.; Leighton, F.A. A History of One Health. *Rev. Sci. Tech.* **2014**, *33*, 413–420.
629. Mackenzie, J.S.; McKinnon, M.; Jeggo, M. One Health: From Concept to Practice. In *Confronting Emerging Zoonoses*; Springer: Tokyo, Japan, 2014; pp. 163–189.
630. Schneider, B.; Balbas-Martinez, V.; Jergens, A.E.; Troconiz, I.F.; Allenspach, K.; Mochel, J.P. Model-Based Reverse Translation between Veterinary and Human Medicine: The One Health Initiative. *CPT Pharmacomet. Syst. Pharmacol.* **2018**, *7*, 65–68.
631. Bontempo, V. Nutrition and Health of Dogs and Cats: Evolution of Petfood. *Vet. Res. Commun.* **2005**, *29*, 45–50
632. Farcas, A.K.; Michel, K.E. Confronting the Problem of Obesity in Dogs and Cats. *Vet. Clin. N. Am.—Small Anim. Pract.* **2016**, *46*, xi–xii.
633. Bartges, J.; Kushner, R.F.; Michel, K.E.; Sallis, R.; Day, M.J. One Health Solutions to Obesity in People and Their Pets. *J. Comp. Pathol.* **2017**, *156*, 326–333.
634. Wakshlag, J.; Loftus, J. Canine and Feline Obesity: A Review of Pathophysiology, Epidemiology, and Clinical Management. *Vet. Med. Res. Rep.* **2014**, *2015*, 49–60.
635. Kapałczyńska, M.; Kolenda, T.; Przybyła, W.; Zajączkowska, M.; Teresiak, A.; Filas, V.; Ibbs, M.; Bliźniak, R.; Łuczewski, Ł.; Lamperska, K. 2D and 3D Cell Cultures—A Comparison of Different Types of Cancer Cell Cultures. *Arch. Med. Sci.* **2018**, *14*, 910–919.

636. Duval, K.; Grover, H.; Han, L.-H.; Mou, Y.; Pegoraro, A.F.; Fredberg, J.; Chen, Z. Modeling Physiological Events in 2D vs. 3D Cell Culture. *Physiology* **2017**, *32*, 266–277.

637. Delie, F.; Rubas, W. A Human Colonic Cell Line Sharing Similarities with Enterocytes as a Model to Examine Oral Absorption: Advantages and Limitations of the Caco-2 Model. *Crit. Rev. Ther. Drug Carr. Syst.* **1997**, *14*, 221–286.

638. Lea, T. Caco-2 Cell Line. In *The Impact of Food Bio-Actives on Gut Health*; Verhoeckx, K., Cotter, P., López-Expósito, I., Kleiveland, C., Lea, T., Mackie, A., Requena, T., Swiatecka, D., Wichers, H., Eds.; Springer: Cham, Switzerland, 2015; pp. 103–111. ISBN 978-3-319-15791-7.

639. Chandra, L.; Borcherding, D.C.; Kingsbury, D.; Atherly, T.; Ambrosini, Y.M.; Bourgois-Mochel, A.; Yuan, W.; Kimber, M.; Qi, Y.; Wang, Q.; et al. Derivation of Adult Canine Intestinal Organoids for Translational Research in Gastroenterology. *BMC Biol.* **2019**, *17*, 33.

640. Schmiedlin-Ren, P.; Thummel, K.E.; Fisher, J.M.; Paine, M.F.; Lown, K.S.; Watkins, P.B. Expression of Enzymatically Active CYP3A4 by Caco-2 Cells Grown on Extracellular Matrix-Coated Permeable Supports in the Presence of 1α,25-Dihydroxyvitamin D3. *Mol. Pharmacol.* **1997**, *51*, 741–754.

641. Anderle, P.; Niederer, E.; Rubas, W.; Hilgendorf, C.; Spahn-Langguth, H.; Wunderli-Allenspach, H.; Merkle, H.P.; Langguth, P. P-Glycoprotein (P-Gp) Mediated Efflux in Caco-2 Cell Monolayers: The Influence of Culturing Conditions and Drug Exposure on P-Gp Expression Levels. *J. Pharm. Sci.* **1998**, *87*, 757–762.

642. Sun, H.; Chow, E.C.; Liu, S.; Du, Y.; Pang, K.S. The Caco-2 Cell Monolayer: Usefulness and Limitations. *Expert. Opin. Drug Metab. Toxicol.* **2008**, *4*, 395–411.

643. Korjamo, T.; Honkakoski, P.; Toppinen, M.-R.; Niva, S.; Reinisalo, M.; Palmgrén, J.J.; Mönkkönen, J. Absorption Properties and P-Glycoprotein Activity of Modified Caco-2 Cell Lines. *Eur. J. Pharm. Sci.* **2005**, *26*, 266–279.

644. Lehmann, R.; Lee, C.M.; Shugart, E.C.; Benedetti, M.; Charo, R.A.; Gartner, Z.; Hogan, B.; Knoblich, J.; Nelson, C.M.; Wilson, K.M. Human Organoids: A New Dimension in Cell Biology. *Mol. Biol. Cell* **2019**, *30*, 1129–1137.

645. Sato, T.; Vries, R.G.; Snippert, H.J.; van de Wetering, M.; Barker, N.; Stange, D.E.; van Es, J.H.; Abo, A.; Kujala, P.; Peters, P.J.; et al. Single Lgr5 Stem Cells Build Crypt-Villus Structures In Vitro without a Mesenchymal Niche. *Nature* **2009**, *459*, 262–265.

646. Gabriel, V.; Zdyrski, C.; Sahoo, D.K.; Dao, K.; Bourgois-Mochel, A.; Kopper, J.; Zeng, X.-L.; Estes, M.K.; Mochel, J.P.; Allenspach, K. Standardization and Maintenance of 3D Canine Hepatic and Intestinal Organoid Cultures for Use in Biomedical Research. *JoVE (J. Vis. Exp.)* **2022**, *179*, e63515.

647. Watanabe, N.; Santostefano, K.E.; Yachnis, A.T.; Terada, N. A Pathologist's Perspective on Induced Pluripotent Stem Cells. *Lab. Investig.* **2017**, *97*, 1126–1132.

648. Sato, T.; Stange, D.E.; Ferrante, M.; Vries, R.G.J.; Van Es, J.H.; Van den Brink, S.; Van Houdt, W.J.; Pronk, A.; Van Gorp, J.; Siersema, P.D.; et al. Long-Term Expansion of Epithelial Organoids from Human Colon,

Adenoma, Adenocarcinoma, and Barrett's Epithelium. *Gastroenterology* **2011**, *141*, 1762–1772.
649. Kim, J.; Koo, B.-K.; Knoblich, J.A. Human Organoids: Model Systems for Human Biology and Medicine. *Nat. Rev. Mol. Cell Biol.* **2020**, *21*, 571–584.
650. Barker, N.; van Es, J.H.; Kuipers, J.; Kujala, P.; van den Born, M.; Cozijnsen, M.; Haegebarth, A.; Korving, J.; Begthel, H.; Peters, P.J.; et al. Identification of Stem Cells in Small Intestine and Colon by Marker Gene Lgr5. *Nature* **2007**, *449*, 1003–1007.
651. Dollé, L.; Theise, N.D.; Schmelzer, E.; Boulter, L.; Gires, O.; van Grunsven, L.A. EpCAM and the Biology of Hepatic Stem/Progenitor Cells. *Am. J. Physiol. Gastrointest. Liver Physiol.* **2015**, *308*, G233–G250. [
652. Zdyrski, C.; Gabriel, V.; Ospina, O.; Wickham, H.; Sahoo, D.K.; Dao, K.; Meza, L.S.A.; Bedos, L.; Honold, S.; Piñeyro, P.; et al. Establishment and Characterization of Novel Canine Organoids with Organ-Specific Physiological Similarity. *bioRxiv* **2022**.
653. Zhao, D.; Farnell, M.B.; Kogut, M.H.; Genovese, K.J.; Chapkin, R.S.; Davidson, L.A.; Berghman, L.R.; Farnell, Y.Z. From Crypts to Enteroids: Establishment and Characterization of Avian Intestinal Organoids. *Poult. Sci.* **2022**, *101*, 101642.
654. Puschhof, J.; Post, Y.; Beumer, J.; Kerkkamp, H.M.; Bittenbinder, M.; Vonk, F.J.; Casewell, N.R.; Richardson, M.K.; Clevers, H. Derivation of Snake Venom Gland Organoids for In Vitro Venom Production. *Nat. Protoc.* **2021**, *16*, 1494–1510.
655. Brandenberg, N.; Hoehnel, S.; Kuttler, F.; Homicsko, K.; Ceroni, C.; Ringel, T.; Gjorevski, N.; Schwank, G.; Coukos, G.; Turcatti, G.; et al. High-

Throughput Automated Organoid Culture via Stem-Cell Aggregation in Microcavity Arrays. *Nat. Biomed. Eng.* **2020**, *4*, 863–874.

656. Wang, M.; Yu, H.; Zhang, T.; Cao, L.; Du, Y.; Xie, Y.; Ji, J.; Wu, J. In-Depth Comparison of Matrigel Dissolving Methods on Proteomic Profiling of Organoids. *Mol. Cell. Proteom.* **2022**, *21*, 100181.
657. Post, Y.; Puschhof, J.; Beumer, J.; Kerkkamp, H.M.; de Bakker, M.A.G.; Slagboom, J.; de Barbanson, B.; Wevers, N.R.; Spijkers, X.M.; Olivier, T.; et al. Snake Venom Gland Organoids. *Cell* **2020**, *180*, 233–247.e21.
658. Elbadawy, M.; Usui, T.; Mori, T.; Tsunedomi, R.; Hazama, S.; Nabeta, R.; Uchide, T.; Fukushima, R.; Yoshida, T.; Shibutani, M.; et al. Establishment of a Novel Experimental Model for Muscle-Invasive Bladder Cancer Using a Dog Bladder Cancer Organoid Culture. *Cancer Sci.* **2019**, *110*, 2806–2821.
659. Bartlett, A.P.; Harman, R.M.; Weiss, J.R.; Van de Walle, G.R. Establishment and Characterization of Equine Mammary Organoids Using a Method Translatable to Other Non-Traditional Model Species. *Development* **2022**, *149*, dev200412.
660. Li, H.; Wang, Y.; Zhang, M.; Wang, H.; Cui, A.; Zhao, J.; Ji, W.; Chen, Y.-G. Establishment of Porcine and Monkey Colonic Organoids for Drug Toxicity Study. *Cell Regen* **2021**, *10*, 32.
661. Chen, T.-C.; Neupane, M.; Chien, S.-J.; Chuang, F.-R.; Crawford, R.B.; Kaminski, N.E.; Chang, C.-C. Characterization of Adult Canine Kidney Epithelial Stem Cells That Give Rise to Dome-Forming Tubular Cells. *Stem Cells Dev.* **2019**, *28*, 1424–1433.
662. Liu, M.; Yu, W.; Jin, J.; Ma, M.; An, T.; Nie, Y.; Teng, C.-B. Copper Promotes Sheep Pancreatic Duct Organoid Growth by Activation of an

Antioxidant Protein 1-Dependent MEK-ERK Pathway. *Am. J. Physiol.—Cell Physiol.* **2020**, *318*, C806–C816.

663. Inaba, A.; Kumaki, S.; Arinaga, A.; Tanaka, K.; Aihara, E.; Yamane, T.; Oishi, Y.; Imai, H.; Iwatsuki, K. Generation of Intestinal Chemosensory Cells from Nonhuman Primate Organoids. *Biochem. Biophys. Res. Commun.* **2021**, *536*, 20–25.
664. Li, J.; Li, J.; Zhang, S.Y.; Li, R.X.; Lin, X.; Mi, Y.L.; Zhang, C.Q. Culture and Characterization of Chicken Small Intestinal Crypts. *Poult. Sci.* **2018**, *97*, 1536–1543.
665. Töpfer, E.; Pasotti, A.; Telopoulou, A.; Italiani, P.; Boraschi, D.; Ewart, M.-A.; Wilde, C. Bovine Colon Organoids: From 3D Bioprinting to Cryopreserved Multi-Well Screening Platforms. *Toxicol. Vitr.* **2019**, *61*, 104606.
666. Stewart, A.S.; Freund, J.M.; Gonzalez, L.M. Advanced Three-Dimensional Culture of Equine Intestinal Epithelial Stem Cells. *Equine Vet. J.* **2018**, *50*, 241–248.
667. Mussard, E.; Pouzet, C.; Helies, V.; Pascal, G.; Fourre, S.; Cherbuy, C.; Rubio, A.; Vergnolle, N.; Combes, S.; Beaumont, M. Culture of Rabbit Caecum Organoids by Reconstituting the Intestinal Stem Cell Niche In Vitro with Pharmacological Inhibitors or L-WRN Conditioned Medium. *Stem Cell Res.* **2020**, *48*, 101980.
668. Gonzalez, L.M.; Williamson, I.; Piedrahita, J.A.; Blikslager, A.T.; Magness, S.T. Cell Lineage Identification and Stem Cell Culture in a Porcine Model for the Study of Intestinal Epithelial Regeneration. *PLoS ONE* **2013**, *8*, e66465.
669. Adegbola, S.; Moore, J.; Sahnan, K.; Tozer, P.; Phillips, R.; Warusavitarne, J.; Faiz, O.; Hart, A. P005 Establishing a Porcine Model to Translate

Anorectal Stem Cell Organoid Models to Elucidate the Aetiology of Perianal Crohn's Fistulae. *J. Crohn's Colitis* **2017**, *11*, S81–S82.

670. Von Furstenberg, R.J.; Gulati, A.S.; Baxi, A.; Doherty, J.M.; Stappenbeck, T.S.; Gracz, A.D.; Magness, S.T.; Henning, S.J. Sorting Mouse Jejunal Epithelial Cells with CD24 Yields a Population with Characteristics of Intestinal Stem Cells. *Am. J. Physiol. Gastrointest. Liver Physiol.* **2011**, *300*, G409–G417.
671. Koltes, D.A.; Gabler, N.K. Characterization of Porcine Intestinal Enteroid Cultures under a Lipopolysaccharide Challenge1. *J. Anim. Sci.* **2016**, *94*, 335–339.
672. Powell, R.H.; Behnke, M.S. WRN Conditioned Media Is Sufficient for In Vitro Propagation of Intestinal Organoids from Large Farm and Small Companion Animals. *Biol. Open* **2017**, *6*, 698–705.
673. Li, L.; Fu, F.; Guo, S.; Wang, H.; He, X.; Xue, M.; Yin, L.; Feng, L.; Liu, P. Porcine Intestinal Enteroids: A New Model for Studying Enteric Coronavirus Porcine Epidemic Diarrhea Virus Infection and the Host Innate Response. *J. Virol.* **2019**, *93*, e01682-18.
674. Acharya, M.; Arsi, K.; Donoghue, A.M.; Liyanage, R.; Rath, N.C. Production and Characterization of Avian Crypt-Villus Enteroids and the Effect of Chemicals. *BMC Vet. Res.* **2020**, *16*, 179.
675. Derricott, H.; Luu, L.; Fong, W.Y.; Hartley, C.S.; Johnston, L.J.; Armstrong, S.D.; Randle, N.; Duckworth, C.A.; Campbell, B.J.; Wastling, J.M.; et al. Developing a 3D Intestinal Epithelium Model for Livestock Species. *Cell Tissue Res.* **2019**, *375*, 409–424.
676. Smith, D.; Price, D.R.G.; Burrells, A.; Faber, M.N.; Hildersley, K.A.; Chintoan-Uta, C.; Chapuis, A.F.; Stevens, M.; Stevenson, K.; Burgess,

S.T.G.; et al. The Development of Ovine Gastric and Intestinal Organoids for Studying Ruminant Host-Pathogen Interactions. *Front. Cell Infect. Microbiol.* **2021**, *11*, 733811.

677. Kardia, E.; Frese, M.; Smertina, E.; Strive, T.; Zeng, X.-L.; Estes, M.; Hall, R.N. Culture and Differentiation of Rabbit Intestinal Organoids and Organoid-Derived Cell Monolayers. *Sci. Rep.* **2021**, *11*, 5401.
678. Tekes, G.; Ehmann, R.; Boulant, S.; Stanifer, M.L. Development of Feline Ileum- and Colon-Derived Organoids and Their Potential Use to Support Feline Coronavirus Infection. *Cells* **2020**, *9*, 2085.
679. Thompson, R.E.; Johnson, A.K.; Dini, P.; Turco, M.Y.; Prado, T.M.; Premanandan, C.; Burton, G.J.; Ball, B.A.; Whitlock, B.K.; Pukazhenthi, B.S. Hormone-Responsive Organoids from Domestic Mare and Endangered Przewalski's Horse Endometrium. *Reproduction* **2020**, *160*, 819–831.
680. Zhou, J.; Li, C.; Liu, X.; Chiu, M.C.; Zhao, X.; Wang, D.; Wei, Y.; Lee, A.; Zhang, A.J.; Chu, H.; et al. Infection of Bat and Human Intestinal Organoids by SARS-CoV-2. *Nat. Med.* **2020**, *26*, 1077–1083.
681. Elbadawy, M.; Kato, Y.; Saito, N.; Hayashi, K.; Abugomaa, A.; Kobayashi, M.; Yoshida, T.; Shibutani, M.; Kaneda, M.; Yamawaki, H.; et al. Establishment of Intestinal Organoid from Rousettus Leschenaultii and the Susceptibility to Bat-Associated Viruses, SARS-CoV-2 and Pteropine Orthoreovirus. *Int. J. Mol. Sci.* **2021**, *22*, 10763.
682. Nantasanti, S.; Spee, B.; Kruitwagen, H.S.; Chen, C.; Geijsen, N.; Oosterhoff, L.A.; van Wolferen, M.E.; Pelaez, N.; Fieten, H.; Wubbolts, R.W.; et al. Disease Modeling and Gene Therapy of Copper Storage Disease in Canine Hepatic Organoids. *Stem Cell Rep.* **2015**, *5*, 895–907.

683. Kruitwagen, H.S.; Oosterhoff, L.A.; Vernooij, I.G.W.H.; Schrall, I.M.; van Wolferen, M.E.; Bannink, F.; Roesch, C.; van Uden, L.; Molenaar, M.R.; Helms, J.B.; et al. Long-Term Adult Feline Liver Organoid Cultures for Disease Modeling of Hepatic Steatosis. *Stem Cell Rep.* **2017**, *8*, 822–830.
684. Wiener, D.J.; Basak, O.; Asra, P.; Boonekamp, K.E.; Kretzschmar, K.; Papaspyropoulos, A.; Clevers, H. Establishment and Characterization of a Canine Keratinocyte Organoid Culture System. *Vet. Dermatol.* **2018**, *29*, 375-e126.
685. Bedos, L.; Wickham, H.; Gabriel, V.; Zdyrski, C.; Allbaugh, R.A.; Sahoo, D.K.; Sebbag, L.; Mochel, J.P.; Allenspach, K. Culture and Characterization of Canine and Feline Corneal Epithelial Organoids: A New Tool for the Study and Treatment of Corneal Diseases. *Front. Vet. Sci.* **2022**, *9*, 1050467.
686. Jung, P.; Sato, T.; Merlos-Suárez, A.; Barriga, F.M.; Iglesias, M.; Rossell, D.; Auer, H.; Gallardo, M.; Blasco, M.A.; Sancho, E.; et al. Isolation and In Vitro Expansion of Human Colonic Stem Cells. *Nat. Med.* **2011**, *17*, 1225–1227.
687. Chua, C.W.; Shibata, M.; Lei, M.; Toivanen, R.; Barlow, L.J.; Bergren, S.K.; Badani, K.K.; McKiernan, J.M.; Benson, M.C.; Hibshoosh, H.; et al. Single Luminal Epithelial Progenitors Can Generate Prostate Organoids in Culture. *Nat. Cell Biol.* **2014**, *16*, 951–961.
688. Tadokoro, T.; Wang, Y.; Barak, L.S.; Bai, Y.; Randell, S.H.; Hogan, B.L.M. IL-6/STAT3 Promotes Regeneration of Airway Ciliated Cells from Basal Stem Cells. *Proc. Natl. Acad. Sci. USA* **2014**, *111*, E3641–E3649.
689. Huch, M.; Gehart, H.; van Boxtel, R.; Hamer, K.; Blokzijl, F.; Verstegen, M.M.A.; Ellis, E.; van Wenum, M.; Fuchs, S.A.; de Ligt, J.; et al. Long-Term Culture of Genome-Stable Bipotent Stem Cells from Adult Human Liver. *Cell* **2015**, *160*, 299–312.

690. Boj, S.F.; Hwang, C.-I.; Baker, L.A.; Chio, I.I.C.; Engle, D.D.; Corbo, V.; Jager, M.; Ponz-Sarvise, M.; Tiriac, H.; Spector, M.S.; et al. Organoid Models of Human and Mouse Ductal Pancreatic Cancer. *Cell* **2015**, *160*, 324–338.
691. Bartfeld, S.; Bayram, T.; van de Wetering, M.; Huch, M.; Begthel, H.; Kujala, P.; Vries, R.; Peters, P.J.; Clevers, H. In Vitro Expansion of Human Gastric Epithelial Stem Cells and Their Responses to Bacterial Infection. *Gastroenterology* **2015**, *148*, 126–136.e6.
692. Jain, R.; Barkauskas, C.E.; Takeda, N.; Bowie, E.J.; Aghajanian, H.; Wang, Q.; Padmanabhan, A.; Manderfield, L.J.; Gupta, M.; Li, D.; et al. Plasticity of Hopx(+) Type I Alveolar Cells to Regenerate Type II Cells in the Lung. *Nat. Commun.* **2015**, *6*, 6727.
693. Kessler, M.; Hoffmann, K.; Brinkmann, V.; Thieck, O.; Jackisch, S.; Toelle, B.; Berger, H.; Mollenkopf, H.-J.; Mangler, M.; Sehouli, J.; et al. The Notch and Wnt Pathways Regulate Stemness and Differentiation in Human Fallopian Tube Organoids. *Nat. Commun.* **2015**, *6*, 8989.
694. Pringle, S.; Maimets, M.; van der Zwaag, M.; Stokman, M.A.; van Gosliga, D.; Zwart, E.; Witjes, M.J.H.; de Haan, G.; van Os, R.; Coppes, R.P. Human Salivary Gland Stem Cells Functionally Restore Radiation Damaged Salivary Glands. *Stem Cells* **2016**, *34*, 640–652.
695. Turco, M.Y.; Gardner, L.; Kay, R.G.; Hamilton, R.S.; Prater, M.; Hollinshead, M.S.; McWhinnie, A.; Esposito, L.; Fernando, R.; Skelton, H.; et al. Trophoblast Organoids as a Model for Maternal–Fetal Interactions during Human Placentation. *Nature* **2018**, *564*, 263–267.
696. Horsley, H.; Dharmasena, D.; Malone-Lee, J.; Rohn, J.L. A Urine-Dependent Human Urothelial Organoid Offers a Potential Alternative to Rodent Models of Infection. *Sci. Rep.* **2018**, *8*, 1238.

697. Gee, K.; Isani, M.A.; Fode, A.; Maselli, K.M.; Zuber, S.M.; Fowler, K.L.; Squillaro, A.I.; Nucho, L.-M.A.; Grikscheit, T.C. Spleen Organoid Units Generate Functional Human and Mouse Tissue-Engineered Spleen in a Murine Model. *Tissue Eng. Part. A* **2020**, *26*, 411–418
698. Rosenbluth, J.M.; Schackmann, R.C.J.; Gray, G.K.; Selfors, L.M.; Li, C.M.-C.; Boedicker, M.; Kuiken, H.J.; Richardson, A.; Brock, J.; Garber, J.; et al. Organoid Cultures from Normal and Cancer-Prone Human Breast Tissues Preserve Complex Epithelial Lineages. *Nat. Commun.* **2020**, *11*, 1711.
699. Liu, Z.; Anderson, J.D.; Deng, L.; Mackay, S.; Bailey, J.; Kersh, L.; Rowe, S.M.; Guimbellot, J.S. Human Nasal Epithelial Organoids for Therapeutic Development in Cystic Fibrosis. *Genes* **2020**, *11*, 603.
700. Ogundipe, V.M.L.; Groen, A.H.; Hosper, N.; Nagle, P.W.K.; Hess, J.; Faber, H.; Jellema, A.L.; Baanstra, M.; Links, T.P.; Unger, K.; et al. Generation and Differentiation of Adult Tissue-Derived Human Thyroid Organoids. *Stem Cell Rep.* **2021**, *16*, 913–925
701. Mollaki, V. Ethical Challenges in Organoid Use. *BioTech* **2021**, *10*, 12.
702. Rock, J.R.; Onaitis, M.W.; Rawlins, E.L.; Lu, Y.; Clark, C.P.; Xue, Y.; Randell, S.H.; Hogan, B.L.M. Basal Cells as Stem Cells of the Mouse Trachea and Human Airway Epithelium. *Proc. Natl. Acad. Sci. USA* **2009**, *106*, 12771–12775
703. Barker, N.; Huch, M.; Kujala, P.; van de Wetering, M.; Snippert, H.J.; van Es, J.H.; Sato, T.; Stange, D.E.; Begthel, H.; van den Born, M.; et al. Lgr5+ve Stem Cells Drive Self-Renewal in the Stomach and Build Long-Lived Gastric Units In Vitro. *Cell Stem Cell* **2010**, *6*, 25–36.
704. Huch, M.; Bonfanti, P.; Boj, S.F.; Sato, T.; Loomans, C.J.M.; Van De Wetering, M.; Sojoodi, M.; Li, V.S.W.; Schuijers, J.; Gracanin, A.; et al.

Unlimited In Vitro Expansion of Adult Bi-Potent Pancreas Progenitors through the Lgr5/R-Spondin Axis. *EMBO J.* **2013**, *32*, 2708–2721

705. Huch, M.; Dorrell, C.; Boj, S.F.; van Es, J.H.; Li, V.S.W.; van de Wetering, M.; Sato, T.; Hamer, K.; Sasaki, N.; Finegold, M.J.; et al. In Vitro Expansion of Single Lgr5+ Liver Stem Cells Induced by Wnt-Driven Regeneration. *Nature* **2013**, *494*, 247–250.
706. Barkauskas, C.E.; Cronce, M.J.; Rackley, C.R.; Bowie, E.J.; Keene, D.R.; Stripp, B.R.; Randell, S.H.; Noble, P.W.; Hogan, B.L.M. Type 2 Alveolar Cells Are Stem Cells in Adult Lung. *J. Clin. Investig.* **2013**, *123*, 3025–3036.
707. Ren, W.; Lewandowski, B.C.; Watson, J.; Aihara, E.; Iwatsuki, K.; Bachmanov, A.A.; Margolskee, R.F.; Jiang, P. Single Lgr5- or Lgr6-Expressing Taste Stem/Progenitor Cells Generate Taste Bud Cells Ex Vivo. *Proc. Natl. Acad. Sci. USA* **2014**, *111*, 16401–16406.
708. DeWard, A.D.; Cramer, J.; Lagasse, E. Cellular Heterogeneity in the Mouse Esophagus Implicates the Presence of a Nonquiescent Epithelial Stem Cell Population. *Cell Rep.* **2014**, *9*, 701–711.
709. Maimets, M.; Rocchi, C.; Bron, R.; Pringle, S.; Kuipers, J.; Giepmans, B.N.G.; Vries, R.G.J.; Clevers, H.; de Haan, G.; van Os, R.; et al. Long-Term In Vitro Expansion of Salivary Gland Stem Cells Driven by Wnt Signals. *Stem Cell Rep.* **2016**, *6*, 150–162.
710. Jamieson, P.R.; Dekkers, J.F.; Rios, A.C.; Fu, N.Y.; Lindeman, G.J.; Visvader, J.E. Derivation of a Robust Mouse Mammary Organoid System for Studying Tissue Dynamics. *Development* **2017**, *144*, 1065–1071.
711. Xie, Y.; Park, E.-S.; Xiang, D.; Li, Z. Long-Term Organoid Culture Reveals Enrichment of Organoid-Forming Epithelial Cells in the Fimbrial Portion of Mouse Fallopian Tube. *Stem Cell Res.* **2018**, *32*, 51–60.

712. Saito, Y.; Onishi, N.; Takami, H.; Seishima, R.; Inoue, H.; Hirata, Y.; Kameyama, K.; Tsuchihashi, K.; Sugihara, E.; Uchino, S.; et al. Development of a Functional Thyroid Model Based on an Organoid Culture System. *Biochem. Biophys. Res. Commun.* **2018**, *497*, 783–789.
713. Santos, C.P.; Lapi, E.; Martínez de Villarreal, J.; Álvaro-Espinosa, L.; Fernández-Barral, A.; Barbáchano, A.; Domínguez, O.; Laughney, A.M.; Megías, D.; Muñoz, A.; et al. Urothelial Organoids Originating from Cd49fhigh Mouse Stem Cells Display Notch-Dependent Differentiation Capacity. *Nat. Commun.* **2019**, *10*, 4407.
714. Pinel, L.; Cyr, D.G. Self-Renewal and Differentiation of Rat Epididymal Basal Cells Using a Novel In Vitro Organoid Model. *Biol. Reprod.* **2021**, *105*, 987–1001.
715. Kar, S.K.; Wells, J.M.; Ellen, E.D.; te Pas, M.F.W.; Madsen, O.; Groenen, M.A.M.; Woelders, H. Organoids: A Promising New in Vitro Platform in Livestock and Veterinary Research. *Vet. Res.* **2021**, *52*, 43.
716. Andersson, L. Domestic Animals as Models for Biomedical Research. *Ups. J. Med. Sci.* **2016**, *121*, 1–11.
717. Axelsson, E.; Ratnakumar, A.; Arendt, M.-L.; Maqbool, K.; Webster, M.T.; Perloski, M.; Liberg, O.; Arnemo, J.M.; Hedhammar, Å.; Lindblad-Toh, K. The Genomic Signature of Dog Domestication Reveals Adaptation to a Starch-Rich Diet. *Nature* **2013**, *495*, 360–364.
718. Beaumont, M.; Blanc, F.; Cherbuy, C.; Egidy, G.; Giuffra, E.; Lacroix-Lamandé, S.; Wiedemann, A. Intestinal Organoids in Farm Animals. *Vet. Res.* **2021**, *52*, 33.

719. Linder, D.E.; Santiago, S.; Halbreich, E.D. Is There a Correlation Between Dog Obesity and Human Obesity? Preliminary Findings of Overweight Status Among Dog Owners and Their Dogs. *Front. Vet. Sci.* **2021**, *8*, 654617.

720. Mahe, M.M.; Aihara, E.; Schumacher, M.A.; Zavros, Y.; Montrose, M.H.; Helmrath, M.A.; Sato, T.; Shroyer, N.F. Establishment of Gastrointestinal Epithelial Organoids. *Curr. Protoc. Mouse Biol.* **2013**, *3*, 217–240

721. Inaba, A.; Arinaga, A.; Tanaka, K.; Endo, T.; Hayatsu, N.; Okazaki, Y.; Yamane, T.; Oishi, Y.; Imai, H.; Iwatsuki, K. Interleukin-4 Promotes Tuft Cell Differentiation and Acetylcholine Production in Intestinal Organoids of Non-Human Primate. *Int. J. Mol. Sci.* **2021**, *22*, 7921.

722. Fujii, M.; Matano, M.; Toshimitsu, K.; Takano, A.; Mikami, Y.; Nishikori, S.; Sugimoto, S.; Sato, T. Human Intestinal Organoids Maintain Self-Renewal Capacity and Cellular Diversity in Niche-Inspired Culture Condition. *Cell Stem Cell* **2018**, *23*, 787–793.e6.

723. Wang, F.; Scoville, D.; He, X.C.; Mahe, M.M.; Box, A.; Perry, J.M.; Smith, N.R.; Lei, N.Y.; Davies, P.S.; Fuller, M.K.; et al. Isolation and Characterization of Intestinal Stem Cells Based on Surface Marker Combinations and Colony-Formation Assay. *Gastroenterology* **2013**, *145*, 383–395.e21.

724. Ahmad, A.A.; Wang, Y.; Gracz, A.D.; Sims, C.E.; Magness, S.T.; Allbritton, N.L. Optimization of 3-D Organotypic Primary Colonic Cultures for Organ-on-Chip Applications. *J. Biol. Eng.* **2014**, *8*, 9.

725. Khalil, H.A.; Lei, N.Y.; Brinkley, G.; Scott, A.; Wang, J.; Kar, U.K.; Jabaji, Z.B.; Lewis, M.; Martín, M.G.; Dunn, J.C.Y.; et al. A Novel Culture System for Adult Porcine Intestinal Crypts. *Cell Tissue Res.* **2016**, *365*, 123–134.

726. Gracz, A.D.; Puthoff, B.J.; Magness, S.T. Identification, Isolation, and Culture of Intestinal Epithelial Stem Cells from Murine Intestine. *Methods Mol. Biol.* **2012**, *879*, 89–107.

727. Von Furstenberg, R.J.; Li, J.; Stolarchuk, C.; Feder, R.; Campbell, A.; Kruger, L.; Gonzalez, L.M.; Blikslager, A.T.; Cardona, D.M.; McCall, S.J.; et al. Porcine Esophageal Submucosal Gland Culture Model Shows Capacity for Proliferation and Differentiation. *Cell Mol. Gastroenterol. Hepatol.* **2017**, *4*, 385–404.

728. Saxena, K.; Blutt, S.E.; Ettayebi, K.; Zeng, X.-L.; Broughman, J.R.; Crawford, S.E.; Karandikar, U.C.; Sastri, N.P.; Conner, M.E.; Opekun, A.R.; et al. Human Intestinal Enteroids: A New Model to Study Human Rotavirus Infection, Host Restriction, and Pathophysiology. *J. Virol.* **2016**, *90*, 43–56.

729. Formeister, E.J.; Sionas, A.L.; Lorance, D.K.; Barkley, C.L.; Lee, G.H.; Magness, S.T. Distinct SOX9 Levels Differentially Mark Stem/Progenitor Populations and Enteroendocrine Cells of the Small Intestine Epithelium. *Am. J. Physiol. Gastrointest. Liver Physiol.* **2009**, *296*, G1108–G1118

730. Kramer, N.; Pratscher, B.; Meneses, A.M.C.; Tschulenk, W.; Walter, I.; Swoboda, A.; Kruitwagen, H.S.; Schneeberger, K.; Penning, L.C.; Spee, B.; et al. Generation of Differentiating and Long-Living Intestinal Organoids Reflecting the Cellular Diversity of Canine Intestine. *Cells* **2020**, *9*, 822.

731. Gabriel, V.; Zdyrski, C.; Sahoo, D.K.; Dao, K.; Bourgois-Mochel, A.; Atherly, T.; Martinez, M.N.; Volpe, D.A.; Kopper, J.; Allenspach, K.; et al. Canine Intestinal Organoids in a Dual-Chamber Permeable Support System. *JoVE (J. Vis. Exp.)* **2022**, *181*, e63612.

732. Ambrosini, Y.M.; Park, Y.; Jergens, A.E.; Shin, W.; Min, S.; Atherly, T.; Borcherding, D.C.; Jang, J.; Allenspach, K.; Mochel, J.P.; et al.

Recapitulation of the Accessible Interface of Biopsy-Derived Canine Intestinal Organoids to Study Epithelial-Luminal Interactions. *PLoS ONE* **2020**, *15*, e0231423.

733. Duzagac, F.; Saorin, G.; Memeo, L.; Canzonieri, V.; Rizzolio, F. Microfluidic Organoids-on-a-chip: Quantum Leap in Cancer Research. *Cancers* **2021**, *13*, 737.

734. Miyoshi, H.; Stappenbeck, T.S. In Vitro Expansion and Genetic Modification of Gastrointestinal Stem Cells in Spheroid Culture. *Nat. Protoc.* **2013**, *8*, 2471–2482.

735. Jung, K.; Eyerly, B.; Annamalai, T.; Lu, Z.; Saif, L.J. Structural Alteration of Tight and Adherens Junctions in Villous and Crypt Epithelium of the Small and Large Intestine of Conventional Nursing Piglets Infected with Porcine Epidemic Diarrhea Virus. *Vet. Microbiol.* **2015**, *177*, 373–378.

736. Hamilton, C.A.; Young, R.; Jayaraman, S.; Sehgal, A.; Paxton, E.; Thomson, S.; Katzer, F.; Hope, J.; Innes, E.; Morrison, L.J.; et al. Development of in Vitro Enteroids Derived from Bovine Small Intestinal Crypts. *Vet. Res.* **2018**, *49*, 54.

737. Co, J.Y.; Margalef-Català, M.; Li, X.; Mah, A.T.; Kuo, C.J.; Monack, D.M.; Amieva, M.R. Controlling Epithelial Polarity: A Human Enteroid Model for Host-Pathogen Interactions. *Cell Rep.* **2019**, *26*, 2509–2520.e4.

738. Kruitwagen, H.S.; Oosterhoff, L.A.; van Wolferen, M.E.; Chen, C.; Nantasanti Assawarachan, S.; Schneeberger, K.; Kummeling, A.; van Straten, G.; Akkerdaas, I.C.; Vinke, C.R.; et al. Long-Term Survival of Transplanted Autologous Canine Liver Organoids in a COMMD1-Deficient Dog Model of Metabolic Liver Disease. *Cells* **2020**, *9*, 410.

739. Van Den Bossche, L.; Schoonenberg, V.A.C.; Burgener, I.A.; Penning, L.C.; Schrall, I.M.; Kruitwagen, H.S.; van Wolferen, M.E.; Grinwis, G.C.M.; Kummeling, A.; Rothuizen, J.; et al. Aberrant Hepatic Lipid Storage and Metabolism in Canine Portosystemic Shunts. *PLoS ONE* **2017**, *12*, e0186491.
740. Wu, X.; Chien, H.; van Wolferen, M.E.; Kruitwagen, H.S.; Oosterhoff, L.A.; Penning, L.C. Reduced FXR Target Gene Expression in Copper-Laden Livers of COMMD1-Deficient Dogs. *Vet. Sci.* **2019**, *6*, 78.
741. Zou, W.Y.; Blutt, S.E.; Crawford, S.E.; Ettayebi, K.; Zeng, X.-L.; Saxena, K.; Ramani, S.; Karandikar, U.C.; Zachos, N.C.; Estes, M.K. Human Intestinal Enteroids: New Models to Study Gastrointestinal Virus Infections. *Methods Mol. Biol.* **2019**, *1576*, 229–247.
742. Haaker, M.W.; Kruitwagen, H.S.; Vaandrager, A.B.; Houweling, M.; Penning, L.C.; Molenaar, M.R.; van Wolferen, M.E.; Oosterhoff, L.A.; Spee, B.; Helms, J.B. Identification of Potential Drugs for Treatment of Hepatic Lipidosis in Cats Using an in Vitro Feline Liver Organoid System. *J. Vet. Intern. Med.* **2020**, *34*, 132–138.
743. Gaush, C.R.; Hard, W.L.; Smith, T.F. Characterization of an Established Line of Canine Kidney Cells (MDCK). *Exp. Biol. Med.* **1966**, *122*, 931–935.
744. Humann-Ziehank, E. Selenium, Copper and Iron in Veterinary Medicine—From Clinical Implications to Scientific Models. *J. Trace Elem. Med. Biol.* **2016**, *37*, 96–103.
745. Agbunag, C.; Lee, K.E.; Buontempo, S.; Bar-Sagi, D. Pancreatic Duct Epithelial Cell Isolation and Cultivation in Two-Dimensional and Three-Dimensional Culture Systems. *Methods Enzym.* **2006**, *407*, 703–710.

746. Zhou, P.; Yang, X.-L.; Wang, X.-G.; Hu, B.; Zhang, L.; Zhang, W.; Si, H.-R.; Zhu, Y.; Li, B.; Huang, C.-L.; et al. A Pneumonia Outbreak Associated with a New Coronavirus of Probable Bat Origin. *Nature* **2020**, *579*, 270–273.
747. Mealey, K.L.; Martinez, S.E.; Villarino, N.F.; Court, M.H. Personalized Medicine: Going to the Dogs? *Hum. Genet.* **2019**, *138*, 467–481.
748. Thompson, R.E.; Meyers, M.A.; Pukazhenthi, B.S.; Hollinshead, F.K. Evaluation of Growth, Viability, and Structural Integrity of Equine Endometrial Organoids Following Cryopreservation. *Cryobiology* **2022**, *104*, 56–62.
749. Thompson, R.E.; Meyers, M.A.; Veeramachaneni, D.N.R.; Pukazhenthi, B.S.; Hollinshead, F.K. Equine Oviductal Organoid Generation and Cryopreservation. *Methods Protoc.* **2022**, *5*, 51.
750. Dundon, M.; Madden, O.; Comizzoli, P. Three-Dimensional Culture of Endometrial Cells from Domestic Cats: A New In Vitro Platform for Assessing Plastic Toxicity. *PLoS ONE* **2019**, *14*, e0217365.
751. Wiener, D.J.; Doherr, M.G.; Müller, E.J.; Suter, M.M.; Welle, M.M. Comparative Assessment of a Canine-Specific Medium to Support Colony Formation from Canine Hair Follicular Keratinocytes. *Vet. Dermatol.* **2015**, *26*, 198-e42.
752. Wiener, D.J.; Studer, I.C.; Brunner, M.A.T.; Hermann, A.; Vincenti, S.; Zhang, M.; Groch, K.R.; Welle, M.M. Characterization of Canine Epidermal Organoid Cultures by Immunohistochemical Analysis and Quantitative PCR. *Vet. Dermatol.* **2021**, *32*, 179-e44.
753. Grego, K.F.; Vieira, S.E.M.; Vidueiros, J.P.; Serapicos, E.d.O.; Barbarini, C.C.; da Silveira, G.P.M.; Rodrigues, F.d.S.; Alves, L.d.C.F.; Stuginski, D.R.; Rameh-de-Albuquerque, L.C.; et al. Maintenance of Venomous Snakes in

Captivity for Venom Production at Butantan Institute from 1908 to the Present: A Scoping History. *J. Venom. Anim. Toxins Incl. Trop. Dis.* **2021**, *27*, e20200068.

754. Gutiérrez, J.M.; León, G.; Burnouf, T. Antivenoms for the Treatment of Snakebite Envenomings: The Road Ahead. *Biologicals* **2011**, *39*, 129–142.
755. Habib, A.G.; Musa, B.M.; Iliyasu, G.; Hamza, M.; Kuznik, A.; Chippaux, J.-P. Challenges and Prospects of Snake Antivenom Supply in Sub-Saharan Africa. *PLoS Negl. Trop. Dis.* **2020**, *14*, e0008374.
756. Chippaux, J.P. Snake-Bites: Appraisal of the Global Situation. *Bull. World Health Organ.* **1998**, *76*, 515–524.
757. O'Brien M. The anatomy of the Achilles tendon. *Foot Ankle Clin*. 2005;10(2):225-238. doi:10.1016/j.fcl.2005.01.011
758. Kayce J. Gross anatomy: Achilles tendon. *Clin Podiatr Med Surg*. 2022;39(3):405-410. doi:10.1016/j.cpm.2022.03.003
759. Duffy DJ, Beamon WL, Chang YJ, Moore GE. Loop modification of the traditional three-loop pulley pattern improves the biomechanical properties and resistance to 3-mm gap formation in a canine common calcanean teno-osseous avulsion model. *Am J Vet Res*. 2022;83(8):ajvr.21.09.0139. doi:10.2460/ajvr.21.09.0139
760. Schulz KS, Ash KJ, Cook JL. Clinical outcomes after common calcanean tendon rupture repair in dogs with a loop-suture tenorrhaphy technique and autogenous leukoreduced platelet-rich plasma. *Vet Surg*. 2019;48(7):1262-1270. doi:10.1111/vsu.13208
761. Beamon WL, Duffy DJ, Chang YJ, Moore GE. Effect of calcanean bone-tunnel orientation for teno-osseous repair in a canine common

calcanean tendon avulsion model. *Vet Surg*. 2022;51(4):688-696. doi:10.1111/vsu.13796

762. O'Brien C, Marr N, Thorpe C. Microdamage in the equine superficial digital flexor tendon. *Equine Vet J*. 2021;53(3):417-430. doi:10.1111/evj.13331
763. Patterson-Kane JC, Rich T. Achilles tendon injuries in elite athletes: lessons in pathophysiology from their equine counterparts. *ILAR J*. 2014;55(1):86-99. doi:10.1093/ilar/ilu004
764. Patterson-Kane JC, Becker DL, Rich T. The pathogenesis of tendon microdamage in athletes: the horse as a natural model for basic cellular research. *J Comp Pathol*. 2012;147(2-3):227-247. doi:10.1016/j.jcpa.2012.05.010
765. Southwood LL, Stashak TS, Kainer RA, Wrigley RH. Desmotomy of the accessory ligament of the superficial digital flexor tendon in the horse with use of a tenoscopic approach to the carpal sheath. *Vet Surg*. 1999;28(2):99-105. doi:10.1053/jvet.1999.0099
766. Gibson KT, Burbidge HM, Anderson BH. Tendonitis of the branches of insertion of the superficial digital flexor tendon in horses. *Aust Vet J*. 1997;75(4):253-256. doi:10.1111/j.1751-0813.1997.tb10091.x
767. Seow D, Islam W, Randall GW, et al. Lower re-rupture rates but higher complication rates following surgical versus conservative treatment of acute achilles tendon ruptures: a systematic review of overlapping meta-analyses. *Knee Surg Sports Traumatol Arthrosc*. 2023;31(8):3528-3540. doi:10.1007/s00167-023-07411-1

768. Chen J, Janney CF, Khalid MA, Panchbhavi VK. Management of insertional Achilles tendinopathy. *J Am Acad Orthop Surg*. 2022;30(10):e751-e759. doi:10.5435/JAAOS-D-21-00679

769. Carmont MR, Knutsson SB, Brorsson A, Karlsson J, Nilsson-Helander K. The release of adhesions improves outcome following minimally invasive repair of Achilles tendon rupture. *Knee Surg Sports Traumatol Arthrosc*. 2022;30(3):1109-1117. doi:10.1007/s00167-021-06767-6

770. Howell MA, McConn TP, Saltrick KR, Catanzariti AR. Calcific insertional Achilles tendinopathy-Achilles repair with flexor hallucis longus tendon transfer: case series and surgical technique. *J Foot Ankle Surg*. 2019;58(2):236-242. doi:10.1053/j.jfas.2018.08.021

771. Levine RS, Pacheco AP, Chope K, García L ópez JM, Gates S, Cos ta LRR. What Is Your Diagnosis? Bilateral SDFT rupture. *J Am Vet Med Assoc*. 2012;241(12):1563-1564. doi:10.2460/javma.241.12.1563

772. Guest DJ, Smith MRW, Allen WR. Equine embryonic stem-like cells and mesenchymal stromal cells have different survival rates and migration patterns following their injection into damaged superficial digital flexor tendon. *Equine Vet J*. 2010;42(7):636-642. doi:10.1111/j.2042-3306.2010.00112.x

773. Geburek F, Mundle K, Conrad S, et al. Tracking of autologous adipose tissue-derived mesenchymal stromal cells with in vivo magnetic resonance imaging and histology after intralesional

treatment of artificial equine tendon lesions-a pilot study. *Stem Cell Res Ther*. 2016;7(1):21. doi:10.1186/s13287-016-0281-8

774. Carvalho AM, Yamada ALM, Golim MA, Álvarez LEC, Hussni C A, Alves ALG. Evaluation of mesenchymal stem cell migration after equine tendonitis therapy. *Equine Vet J*. 2014;46(5):635-638. doi:10.1111/evj.12173
775. Godwin EE, Young NJ, Dudhia J, Beamish IC, Smith RKW. Impl antation of bone marrow-derived mesenchymal stem cells demonstrates improved outcome in horses with overstrain injury of the superficial digital flexor tendon. *Equine Vet J*. 2012;44(1):25-32. doi:10.1111/j.2042-3306.2011.00363.x
776. Lang HM, Schnabel LV, Cassano JM, Fortier LA. Effect of needle diameter on the viability of equine bone marrow derived mesenchymal stem cells. *Vet Surg*. 2017;46(5):731-737. doi:10.1111/vsu.12639
777. Williams LB, Russell KA, Koenig JB, Koch TG. Aspiration, but not injection, decreases cultured equine mesenchymal stromal cell viability. *BMC Vet Res*. 2016;12(1):45. doi:10.1186/s12917-016-0671-2
778. Rowland AL, Burns ME, Levine GJ, Watts AE. Preparation technique affects recipient immune targeting of autologous mesenchymal stem cells. *Front Vet Sci*. 2021;8:724041. doi:10.3389/fvets.2021.724041
779. Pilgrim CR, McCahill KA, Rops JG, Dufour JM, Russell KA, Koc h TG. A review of fetal bovine serum in the culture of mesenchymal stromal cells and potential alternatives for veterinary

medicine. *Front Vet Sci*. 2022;9:859025. doi:10.3389/fvets.2022.859025

780. Naskou MC, Tyma JF, Gordon J, et al. Equine platelet lysate gel: a matrix for mesenchymal stem cell delivery. *Stem Cells Dev*. 2022;31(17-18):569-578. doi:10.1089/scd.2022.0097

781. Bohannon LK, Owens SD, Walker NJ, Carrade DD, Galuppo LD, Borjesson DL. The effects of therapeutic concentrations of gentamicin, amikacin and hyaluronic acid on cultured bone marrow-derived equine mesenchymal stem cells. *Equine Vet J*. 2013;45(6):732-736. doi:10.1111/evj.12045

782. Schnabel LV, Fortier LA, McIlwraith CW, Nobert KM. Therapeuti c use of stem cells in horses: which type, how, and when? *Vet J*. 2013;197(3):570-577. doi:10.1016/j.tvjl.2013.04.018

783. Sole A, Spriet M, Padgett KA, et al. Distribution and persistence of technetium-99 hexamethyl propylene amine oxime-labelled bone marrow-derived mesenchymal stem cells in experimentally induced tendon lesions after intratendinous injection and regional perfusion of the equine distal limb. *Equine Vet J*. 2013;45(6):726-731. doi:10.1111/evj.12063

784. Becerra P, Valdés V ázquez MA, Dudhia J, et al. Distribution of injected technetium(99m)-labeled mesenchymal stem cells in horses with naturally occurring tendinopathy. *J Orthop Res*. 2013;31(7):1096-1102. doi:10.1002/jor.22338

785. Ma S, Xie N, Li W, Yuan B, Shi Y, Wang Y. Immunobiology of mesenchymal stem cells. *Cell Death Differ*. 2014;21(2):216-225. doi:10.1038/cdd.2013.158

786. Noronha NC, Mizukami A, Caliári-Oliveira C, et al. Priming approaches to improve the efficacy of mesenchymal stromal cell-based therapies. *Stem Cell Res Ther*. 2019;10(1):131. doi:10.1186/s13287-019-1224-y

787. Li M, Jiang Y, Hou Q, Zhao Y, Zhong L, Fu X. Potential pre-activation strategies for improving therapeutic efficacy of mesenchymal stem cells: current status and future prospects. *Stem Cell Res Ther*. 2022;13(1):146. doi:10.1186/s13287-022-02822-2

788. Koch DW, Berglund AK, Messenger KM, Gilbertie JM, Ellis IM, Schnabel LV. Interleukin-1β in tendon injury enhances reparative gene and protein expression in mesenchymal stem cells. *Front Vet Sci*. 2022;9:963759. doi:10.3389/fvets.2022.963759

789. Berglund AK, Schnabel LV. Allogeneic major histocompatibility complex-mismatched equine bone marrow-derived mesenchymal stem cells are targeted for death by cytotoxic anti-major histocompatibility complex antibodies. *Equine Vet J*. 2017;49(4):539-544. doi:10.1111/evj.12647

790. Schnabel LV, Pezzanite LM, Antczak DF, Felippe MJB, Fortier LA. Equine bone marrow-derived mesenchymal stromal cells are heterogeneous in MHC class II expression and capable of inciting an immune response in vitro. *Stem Cell Res Ther*. 2014;5(1):13. doi:10.1186/scrt402

791. Rowland AL, Miller D, Berglund A, et al. Cross-matching of allogeneic mesenchymal stromal cells eliminates recipient immune targeting. *Stem Cells Transl Med*. 2021;10(5):694-710. doi:10.1002/sctm.20-0435

792. Berglund AK, Fisher MB, Cameron KA, Poole EJ, Schnabel LV. Transforming growth factor-β2 downregulates major histocompatibility complex (MHC) I and MHC II surface expression on equine bone marrow-derived mesenchymal stem cells without altering other phenotypic cell surface markers. *Front Vet Sci*. 2017;4:84. doi:10.3389/fvets.2017.00084
793. Berglund AK, Long JM, Robertson JB, Schnabel LV. TGF-β2 reduces the cell-mediated immunogenicity of equine MHC-mismatched bone marrow-derived mesenchymal stem cells without altering immunomodulatory properties. *Front Cell Dev Biol*. 2021;9:628382. doi:10.3389/fcell.2021.628382
794. Koch DW, Schnabel LV, Ellis IM, Bates RE, Berglund AK. TGF-β2 enhances expression of equine bone marrow-derived mesenchymal stem cell paracrine factors with known associations to tendon healing. *Stem Cell Res Ther*. 2022;13(1):477. doi:10.1186/s13287-022-03172-9
795. Pacini S, Spinabella S, Trombi L, et al. Suspension of bone marrow-derived undifferentiated mesenchymal stromal cells for repair of superficial digital flexor tendon in race horses. *Tissue Eng*. 2007;13(12):2949-2955. doi:10.1089/ten.2007.0108
796. Salz RO, Elliott CRB, Zuffa T, Bennet ED, Ahern BJ. Treatment of racehorse superficial digital flexor tendonitis: a comparison of stem cell treatments to controlled exercise rehabilitation in 213 cases. *Equine Vet J*. Published online January 16, 2023. doi:10.1111/evj.13922

797. Van den Boom NAC, Winters M, Haisma HJ, Moen MH. Efficacy of stem cell therapy for tendon disorders: a systematic review. *Orthop J Sports Med*. 2020;8(4):2325967120915857. doi:10.1177/2325967120915857

798. Thorpe CT, Godinho MSC, Riley GP, Birch HL, Clegg PD, Screen HRC. The interfascicular matrix enables fascicle sliding and recovery in tendon, and behaves more elastically in energy storing tendons. *J Mech Behav Biomed Mater*. 2015; 52:85-94. doi:10.1016/j.jmbbm.2015.04.009

799. Myhrvold SB, Brouwer EF, Andresen TKM, et al. Nonoperative or surgical treatment of acute Achilles' tendon rupture. *N Engl J Med*. 2022;386(15):1409-1420. doi:10.1056/NEJMoa2108447

About Authors

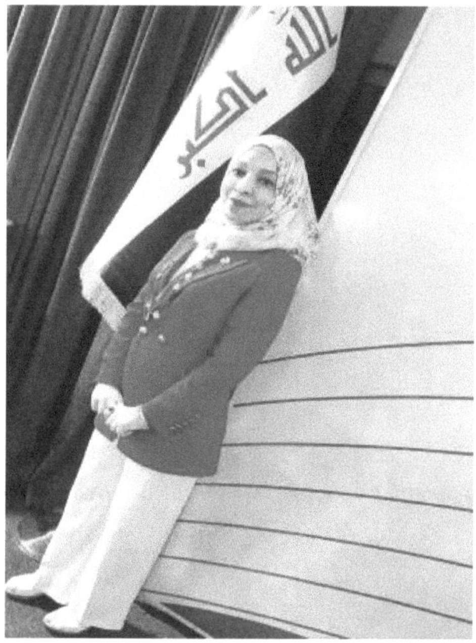

Assist. Prof. Dr. Zainab A.SHEHAB

Department of physiology, pharmacology and Biochemistry, College of veterinary medicine,

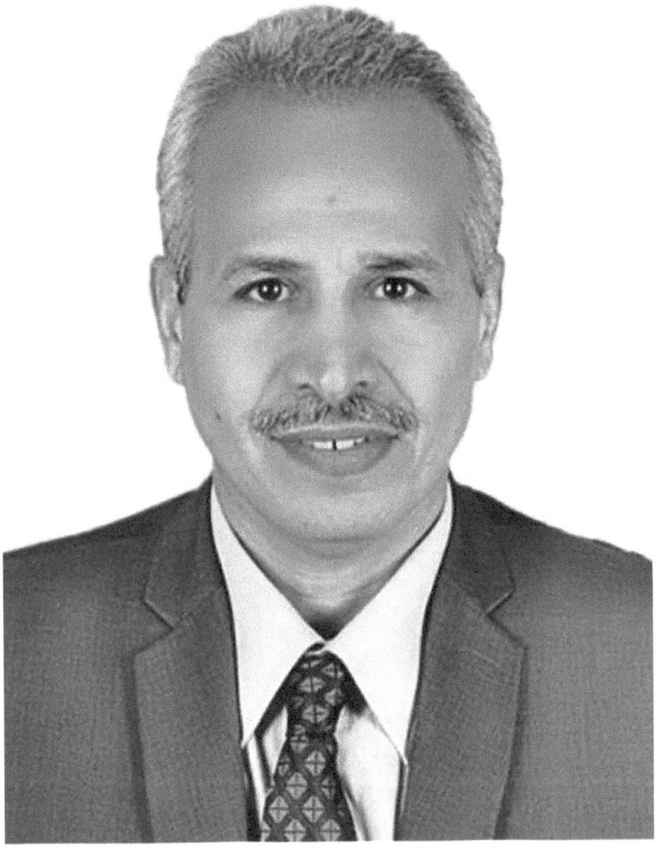

Prof. Dr. Mohamed Abdel-Raheem Ali Abdel-Raheem

Professor of Entomology (Biological Control)

Pests & Plant Protection Department

Agricultural and Biological Research Institute

National Research Centre.

33rd ElBohouth St., Dokki, Cairo, Egypt.

Email: abdelraheem_nrc@hotmail.com,

abdelraheem_nrc@yahoo.com

Mobile: (+2) 01155527583 - (+2) 01009580797

Prof. Dr. Mohamed Abdel-Raheem Ali Abdel-Raheem, Prof. of Entomology (Biological Control), Pests & Plant Protection Department, Agricultural and Biological Research Institute, National Research Centre, Cairo, Egypt. Published publications (281) papers (82), Books and Book chapters (199), (Scopus) h-index (10), Citations (286), (Google Scholar) h-index (19) , Citations (916), (Web of Science) Publications (9), h-index (5), Citations (51), Research Gate, h-index (14), Citations (621), Reviewers in International Journals (132), Reviewed articles in Biological Control (747), Editor in Chief in Journal (6), Editorial board in Journals (32), Associated Editor in Chief in Journal (5), conference Attended (27), workshop Attended (292), Symposium Attended (176), Forum Attended (4), Prize (4), Attended Others (30), Projects As PI and member (19), Training courses For Agric. Engineering (20), Training courses For Students of University (8), attending Trainees courses (19), TV & Radio (26), Supervisor on Ph.D. thesis (1), Committee Ph.D. thesis (2), and member in scientific Foundation (13).

National Research Centre. 33rd ElBohouth St., Dokki, Cairo, Egypt. Email Address: abdelraheem_nrc@hotmail.com, abdelraheem_nrc@yahoo.com, ma.abdel-raheem@nrc.sci.eg, Mobile Phone: (+2) 01155527583 – (+2) 01009580797

Scopus Author ID : 55220661700

https://www.scopus.com/authid/detail.uri?authorId=55220661700

http://scholar.google.com/citations?hl=en&user=gBtssEgAAAAJ

https://orcid.org/my-orcid?orcid=0000-0001-9240-064X

https://www.webofscience.com/wos/author/searchAbdel-Raheem, Mohamed Abdel-Raheem Ali - Web of Science Core Collection

- https://www.researchgate.net/profile/Mohamed_Abdel-Raheem4/publications?sorting=recentlyAdded
- http://livedna.org/20.16018
- http://www.resarcherid.com/rid/R-6264-2017
- https://www.webofscience.com/wos/author/record/R-6264-2017
- https://www.youtube.com/attribution_link?a=NsH2xGv9mY8&u=%2Fwatch%3Fv%3Dsb46rBG8-Mc%26feature%3Dshare
- https://youtu.be/Ub8djW0tggo
- https://m.facebook.com/story.php?story_fbid=492907069288338&id=100076011247165
- https://youtu.be/dOujUAZmTdw
- https://m.facebook.com/story.php?story_fbid=492907069288338&id=100076011247165
- https://fb.watch/gPGrDuzZFX/
- https://www.youtube.com/watch?si=4UfyQaeHVLPiVR5J&v=nXV4NT-no7o&feature=youtu.be
- https://www.youtube.com/watch?v=sRH44W6TbcQ
- https://youtu.be/uq9Qj3AEBHk?si=ymaX06huG2AXJESu

Dr. Hind A. A. Alahmed

Department of physiology, pharmacology and Biochemistry, College of veterinary medicine, University of Basrah, Iraq

Kolibri 360 GmbH
Ferdinand-Jühlke-Straße 7
99095 Erfurt, Deutschland
produktsicherheit@kolibri360.de

Druck:
CPI Druckdienstleistungen GmbH
im Auftrag der
Kolibri 360 GmbH
Ferdinand-Jühlke-Str. 7
99095 Erfurt